CELLULAR
AWAKENING
How your body holds and creates light

CELLULAR
AWAKENING

How your body holds and creates light

BARBARA WREN

HAY HOUSE

Carlsbad, California • New York City • London
Sydney •Johannesburg • Vancouver • New Delhi

First published and distributed in the United Kingdom by:
Hay House UK Ltd, Astley House, 33 Notting Hill Gate, London W11 3JQ
Tel: +44 (0)20 3675 2450; Fax: +44 (0)20 3675 2451; www.hayhouse.co.uk

Published and distributed in the United States of America by:
Hay House Inc., PO Box 5100, Carlsbad, CA 92018-5100
Tel: (1) 760 431 7695 or (800) 654 5126
Fax: (1) 760 431 6948 or (800) 650 5115; www.hayhouse.com

Published and distributed in Australia by:
Hay House Australia Ltd, 18/36 Ralph St, Alexandria NSW 2015
Tel: (61) 2 9669 4299; Fax: (61) 2 9669 4144; www.hayhouse.com.au

Published and distributed in the Republic of South Africa by:
Hay House SA (Pty) Ltd, PO Box 990, Witkoppen 2068
info@hayhouse.co.za; www.hayhouse.co.za

Published and distributed in India by:
Hay House Publishers India, Muskaan Complex, Plot No.3, B-2,
Vasant Kunj, New Delhi 110 070
Tel: (91) 11 4176 1620; Fax: (91) 11 4176 1630; www.hayhouse.co.in

Distributed in Canada by:
Raincoast Books, 2440 Viking Way, Richmond, B.C. V6V 1N2
Tel: (1) 604 448 7100; Fax: (1) 604 270 7161; www.raincoast.com

The information given in this book should not be treated as a substitute for professional
medical advice; always consult a medical practitioner. Any use of information in this book
is at the reader's discretion and risk. Neither the author nor the publisher can be held
responsible for any loss, claim or damage arising out of the use, or misuse, of the suggestions
made, the failure to take medical advice or for any material on third party websites.

A catalogue record for this book is available from the British Library.

ISBN: 978-1-84850-103-4

Printed and bound in Great Britain by TJ International, Padstow, Cornwall.

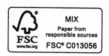

MIX
Paper from
responsible sources
FSC
www.fsc.org   FSC® C013056

'The human body is the best portrayal of the universe in miniature. Whatever does not exist in the human body cannot be found in the universe, and whatever exists in the universe can be found in the human body.'

Mahatma Gandhi

*To my grandmother, Jane, who taught me
from a very young age that it was love that
made the world go round.*

Contents

Foreword

The first time I met Barbara Wren, there was something about her energy that was instantly likeable. She talks very seriously about health and healing, but always with a twinkle in her eye. What is so wonderful and refreshing about her teaching is that it connects you with a deep inner knowing. There is a consistency and sense to everything she says that resonates with certain feelings that we have all had in the past but perhaps dismissed. She speaks with integrity because she lives her philosophy day to day. Although when I met her I already had a deep knowledge of health and healing, her discussion of how we hold and utilize light inspired me to study with her. Over the course of two years I learned about the body and its connection to the greater universe in a way that took me deep inside myself. Barbara's basic philosophy revolves around personal responsibility and empowerment, and it is this that makes her work so appealing. She invites everyone she teaches to take control of their lives and to embark on a journey to deeper levels of health, happiness and freedom.

If you have been suffering from ill health, whether for a long or short time, this book will connect you to an understanding of yourself that will enable you to find genuine long-term healing. If you are already on a path of healing, you will discover tools that can dramatically speed up the process and bring about swift and powerful change. When I discovered Barbara's teachings, I had enjoyed a deep quality of health and happiness for many years. You might think that this meant she had little to offer me, but nothing could be further from the truth. I tested out her teachings, I researched the many eminent doctors, scientists and philosophers who inspired her, and the journey it took me on has been truly life changing. I have had so many shifts in consciousness and have made so many new connections in my understanding of health and healing that I continue to be both thrilled and amazed by the power of the process.

Barbara not only shares her philosophy but also has over three decades of deep experience of helping people become whole and empowered in their lives. Over that time she has accumulated a wonderful 'medicine bag' of tools that she uses with great efficiency to facilitate positive change in her own life and the lives of the many people who have over the years sought out her wisdom. In this book she shares each of those tools with you and invites you to try them out for yourself to experience their unique power. I strongly recommend that you do. Their simplicity and power make them life changing. Imagine owning a wonderful car and suddenly discovering that you had inside you all the knowledge you ever needed to maintain that car in perfect running order. Add to this all the tools you need to achieve this and you'd never need to take it to a mechanic again.

Barbara likens the body to a vehicle and shows each of us how we can uncover the knowledge that is hidden within each and every one of us to keep that vehicle in the very best of condition.

Over the many years that I have been studying, I have found Barbara's teachings amongst the most powerful that I have ever met. She is a true visionary. Having applied and tested her teachings in my own life and in the lives of clients, I can say with full assurance that this stuff works. Don't take my word for it, though – test it out for yourself. I think you'll be amazed by how different you can feel.

Barbara also has a philosophy that is so pertinent to the times in which we are living. She helps people to connect with who they really are and to feel truly empow-ered. What she says makes sense and presents a new way of looking at health and healing. This book takes away the mystery of how to be healthy and places you firmly in charge of who you are and where you are going. Barbara does not ask you to believe what she says but to feel for yourself the resonance of truth. We are each born with an inner knowing of who we are and what our purpose is, but so many of us have forgotten this and become sidetracked by life. Barbara challenges each of us to take full responsibility for our own lives and to remember just how wonderful and amazing we really are. We are beings that thrive on light and have the potential to hold light within and around every cell in our bodies. This gives a whole new meaning to the idea of enlightenment and opens the mind up to new possibilities. So sit down, relax and prepare to uncover your amazing potential. **Andy Baggott**

Acknowledgements

To my children and grandchildren, who have willingly or otherwise been such a huge part of my learning. I would like to say a special thank you to my son Benjamin, who has worked beside me throughout within a college that continues to challenge current thinking.

Appreciation goes to Andy Baggott for his inspirational and intuitive ghostwriting and to him and his partner Debbie for their constant positive and magical support throughout the creation of this book.

Thanks to Michelle Pilley and all at Hay House for giving me this wonderful opportunity to express myself at a time when teaching through a college is becoming more restricted.

PART I

How our Amazing Body Resonates with the Universe

CHAPTER I

CONNECTING WITH INNER WISDOM

We are living in the most exciting of times. The Earth is going through significant changes and our galaxy is moving into a new astrological age. New discoveries are being made in science and technology almost on a daily basis. New species are being discovered in the natural world, old knowledge that appeared lost is re-emerging and there is a vast amount of new information at our fingertips. We are communicating with each other at a level never before achieved. Information is now more freely available to us than it has ever been and it seems as if there is a flood of new ideas, new scientific discoveries and new news. Each day we know more than we did the day before. Each day our consciousness is expanded. We wake every morning with new questions in our minds, whether we are consciously aware of them or not. For some people the questions are mundane, but more and more people are asking deeper questions about who we really are and what life is all about.

Every day we receive fresh information from the media, some of which might perhaps hold the answers we are seeking. But how do we sift through all this information and decide what is relevant to us and what is not? More important, how do we discern what is true and what is false? So much of the information is contradictory, especially when it comes to our health. One day chocolate is good for you, the next day it is bad for you. One day red wine might help you live longer by guarding you against heart disease, the next day it might shorten your life by making you more susceptible to liver disease. It is hard to know just what to believe.

In the West we have been subjected to a most enormous con. We have been taught that if we require wisdom and knowledge, we need to look outside ourselves. We have been taught that the vital information is held in libraries, in universities and in the minds of other people. We have never been taught that we can look within. Although in recent years many people have begun a journey back to themselves through meditation, yoga and other Eastern practices, there has still been a tendency to seek other people to tell us how to be ourselves. However, every time we go outside ourselves to seek our wisdom, it immediately becomes someone else's wisdom and not our own. We are not able to contribute our own uniqueness, our own wisdom, to the universal picture, to the greater whole. And we need to live our uniqueness because this is what creates the order of the greater whole. As soon as we cease to look inside and instead look outside, there is mediocrity, standardization and control across the globe.

The answer to any question you might ask is to be found within you. The truth is not 'out there' but inside your own amazing being, for you are much more than you could possibly imagine.

We are not separate, isolated individuals but multi-dimensional, interconnected beings of light living in an inter-connected universe. What unfolds around us has a direct and tangible influence on our body, and likewise how we live has a direct effect on the universe. We are vibrational beings living in a vibrational universe that at its most funda-mental level is composed of a combination of energy and consciousness. We each create our own reality through our consciousness, but it is the body that is the vehicle for that consciousness. If the body is not balanced then conscious-ness cannot be fully expressed. As a result we become more contracted and in turn our world becomes more contracted to us.

There is nothing wrong with the universe itself; it is in perfect balance. This is not a static balance but a state of dynamic equilibrium, because the universe is forever flowing and expanding. It is conscious and knows how to balance itself so that continued expansion is possible. It holds within its fabric the understanding of how to achieve that balance. This understanding is called *universal wisdom* and it is the wisdom of harmony. Universal wisdom permeates everything. It is within all matter, every planet, every living thing and every subatomic particle.

Likewise there is nothing wrong with Mother Earth, for she is part of this conscious universe and she too holds the wisdom of how to remain in balance. No matter what we as humans do to this planet, nature always brings things back into harmony. Where we have scoured the Earth or polluted it, over time nature replenishes and cleanses. This is the great power that allows for the continuation of life.

Rudolf Steiner said that if we want to heal ourselves, we must first heal the Earth, and indeed there is much wisdom in these words. Mother Earth is a bountiful provider and the more care and attention we give to her, the more she gives in return. When allowed to, she provides everything we need in its most potent and vital form to facilitate our wellbeing and our continued expansion.

It is our natural condition to be at one with the Earth and universe. The sages of old understood this. When our microcosm, the energies we hold at a cellular level, matches the macrocosm, the world outside our body, there is nothing that we cannot do. We were born to dream and then through our expanding consciousness to make those dreams reality. We were born to have great ideas and then make those ideas real. What kind of life do you want to live? What kind of experiences would you like to have and, more important, what kind of experiences would you like to avoid? Everything is possible for us when we live in harmony with the macrocosm. This is the true meaning of human potential.

We hear relatively little these days about fulfilling our

potential and what we do hear paints a much diluted picture. To fulfil your potential in modern society means things like achieving good grades at school, getting a good job, owning your own property, being financially solvent and saving for your retirement. And at the back of these ideas lies the fear of not being able to achieve this potential because of ill health.

As children we all have dreams of what we want to do when we grow up, but as we get older we are usually taught to compromise our dreams, to wake up and learn to live in the 'real world'. In fact the truth is that we have been taught to fall asleep and become disconnected from what life is really about.

There is only one thing that will ever stop you from doing what you really want to and that is fear. So much attention is given to perpetuating fear in our modern society, for it is a most effective way to control the masses. We fear poverty, ill health, war and terrorism, and governments make sure we continue to give our attention to these things by telling us that they are declaring war on all that we fear. But fear is never released through fighting, because war of any kind only serves to promote more fear. Perhaps it is time for us to choose to give our attention to what we want rather than what we don't want.

Can you imagine how wonderful it must feel to have no fear? Wouldn't it be great to understand your own body so well that you could quickly and efficiently bring it into balance and harmony? Wouldn't it be fine to be able to live in full abundance on every level, to live the life of your dreams?

If we can learn to release our fear and connect to our

inner wisdom there is truly nothing that we cannot do. We are told that we use only 10 per cent of our brain. Just imagine what we could achieve if we could illuminate the other 90 per cent. Where would we go then in our development as a race and what would the world be like if we were able to sense it in this more expanded way?

Happiness, health and freedom are the birthright of every person on this planet and are achievable by every person on this planet. No matter where you are in your life, no matter what your state of health or ill health, you have the potential to find happiness, health and freedom.

As we learn to illuminate our potential we become what to others might appear a walking miracle. No longer is any disease 'incurable', for we understand that all illness is totally and unequivocally curable from within, without exception. No longer do we dread what the future holds, for we walk forever infused with an inner knowing that we are masters of our own destiny. This is what human potential is really about. It is about lighting up our lives in ever more wonderful and exciting ways. It is about daring to dream and then walking towards those dreams with open arms, free of fear. It is about being who we really are, who we know in our heart we were always meant to be.

The biggest stress that we can experience is not being able to be who we are. In order to be ourselves we need to maintain the right connections with the Earth and the universe, to be in balance with all that is around us. This means matching our microcosm, the vibration we hold at a cellular level, with the macrocosm, the world about us.

Something that has been so negated in the teachings

and reductionism of the West is the fact that we have a body. I refer to this body as our 'vehicle'. It is this vehicle that has the ability to manifest from within itself everything that is represented in the outer universe. But it is only when we are in a state of balance and harmony that we can truly tap into universal wisdom and make it our own at a cellular level. So much of our work together in this book will be about how to prepare our body, our vehicle, to receive and hold universal wisdom. How to treat the vehicle in order to be able to do this seems to me to be the most important aspect of health.

When we talk about health, we are not talking about a lack of symptoms but a deep connectedness to who we are and our place within the universe. This connectedness needs to unfold at a physical, emotional and spiritual level. Currently in the West these three aspects are not united but kept very separate. At one end you have confusing and often contradictory information about how to maintain the physical body through nutrition, while at the other end you have spiritual practices. As for our emotions, they receive precious little attention in any productive way. If you are having emotional problems you might at best see a therapist and at worst be prescribed a suppressive drug that further cuts you off from who you really are. But it is our emotional journey that brings the physical and spiritual together in unity. How you feel emotionally is without doubt the best possible indicator you have of whether you are heading towards harmony or disharmony. It is your guide to the fulfilment of your dreams. When you feel good, you know you are heading in the right direction. When you feel bad, you know that you are heading away from the life you really want. If you consistently seek out better feelings, your vehicle will transport you on the adventure of a lifetime to places beyond your dreams.

When we talk about connecting with our feelings, we are not talking about contacting our inner anger, guilt, disappointment and fear, we are talking about connecting both with our inner wisdom and with the macrocosm. Our planet goes through many cycles of change and we are intrinsically linked to these cycles. Learning to be aware of and feel these changing cycles allows us to bring ourselves into harmonious union with Mother Earth.

Whether we are aware of them or not, we feel every change in the Earth at a cellular level. When we can navigate these changes successfully, all is well, but when we fall out of harmony with these changes then dis-ease is manifested. We are also intrinsically linked to the changes that occur outside our planet. Everybody knows that the moon has a strong influence on the water on this planet but what many have forgotten is that we are predominantly made up of water and so the moon also has a strong influence upon us.

All of the planets in our solar system exert their influences upon us as they go through their orbits, affecting different organs and minerals within our vehicle. I have known this fact for many years and it has proved very useful, especially when trying to connect people with what is unfolding within their own vehicles at different times.

For example, I had a gentleman come to see me as a patient and during my consultation with him I asked him if he suffered from headaches. He said that he had in the past but after seeing one of my former students, who suggested he drank four pints (two and a half litres) of water a day, the headaches had disappeared. He had not had a headache since then until very recently, when he had had an unexpected migraine. I stopped him at this point and said that I felt I knew the exact day on which that would have occurred. I told him the day and he was amazed that I was correct. I was able to do this because I was aware of several interconnected facts. I knew that migraines and the liver were intrinsically linked and that the planet Mars had a strong energetic influence upon the liver. I also knew that in its orbit around the sun Mars had recently come into close proximity to the Earth and so I chose the day when it had been at its closest and therefore had its strongest influence. If this patient had been aware of this information prior to seeing me, he might well have been able to support his liver with an appropriate technique (see *Chapter 9*) and so avoided experiencing the migraine. Even if he had been unable to do this, the migraine would have no longer been an unexpected and unexplainable occurrence.

Nothing happens in the universe by chance; everything is part of an unfolding and interconnected process.

A Significant Time for our Planet

Our planet is going through three particular changes at the moment that seem to me to be highly significant when you consider how we are connected to Mother Earth.

First, the Earth's magnetic field is becoming steadily weaker. Scientists surmise that this is a sign that the magnetic poles are likely to reverse in the near future, just as they have many times in the past. If you just consider the facts that our blood is composed of a high concentration of iron and that iron is influenced magnetically, this change in the Earth must also effect a change in us. It feels to me as if this reduction in magnetic strength is giving us the potential to think more expansively and freely. It is as if we are no longer being held in old thought patterns but have the opportunity to think in new and exciting ways. Old paradigms are crumbling both in the scientific and spiritual worlds. Quantum physics is showing that science and spirituality have much common ground, whereas in the past they appeared to be poles apart.

Secondly, the Earth's speed of vibration, its resonance, is increasing. Everything in the universe vibrates with energy, and the Earth is no different. This vibration, known as the Schumann Resonance, has been steadily increasing over the past 40 years. The planet is literally speeding up. Our hypothalamus and pituitary glands tune into this vibration and within each of our cells there are receptors in the protein channels that pick up all the vibrations from outside. So we are intimately connected to this change in vibration and more and more people are becoming intuitively aware of it as well. So many people that I meet talk about having the sense of time speeding up and I believe this is a direct effect of this vibrational increase. I also believe that we have the potential to increase our own vibration, to achieve higher states of awareness and connectedness, and in doing so to gain access to deeper levels of our inner wisdom.

The third significant change is that we are seeing a dramatic increase in photon activity, both in our sun and from outside our solar system. Photons are subatomic particles of light, so this means that there is a dramatic increase in the light available within our solar system and on our planet.

We are about to fully enter what is called 'the photon belt', a ring of photons. Just as our planet revolves around a star, the sun, so our solar system revolves around a great star. This great circuit takes approximately 26,000 years and is elliptical, meaning that at certain times we are a relatively long way away from our great star and at other times quite close. If you divide this orbit into 12 equal segments as a means of marking the passage of time and assign the signs of the zodiac to each twelfth, the times when we are closest to our great star correspond to the times of Leo and Aquarius. This is what is meant by the 'Age of Aquarius'. These times are also when we pass through the photon belt. In 2012 we will fully enter it for the first time in 11,000 years, but we are already feeling its influence.

Entering the photon belt marks the dawn of a new era lasting approximately 2,100 years when we are bathed in a much greater number of photons. In the past, times of high photon activity have coincided with great leaps forward in our thinking and development, and we are now living in another time of dramatic progress and development, both intellectually and spiritually. One only needs to look at the changes that have taken place since the emergence of the microchip to realize this. The challenge for us is to match the changes occurring in the macrocosm within our own microcosm. We need to have our vehicle in a state of heightened receptiveness in order to take full advantage of these macrocosmic shifts. We need to be open in our cells and in our mind.

Looking at the Body as a Test Tube

As well as looking at the body as a vehicle, another useful analogy is to look at it as a test tube. If we were a scientist conducting experiments in the test tube, the conditions within it would have a great influence upon the outcome of those experiments. Indeed, we know that changes in the levels of light availability, hydration, pH and temperature all have dramatic effects on the body.

Light is of great importance because it connects everything in the universe, including every single cell in our body. So light availability and the body's own ability to store and utilize light become very important if we are to connect with and illuminate our inner wisdom.

Hydration is also vital. In the next chapter we will see how as soon as our body becomes dehydrated, the condition of every cell membrane is changed. I refer to the cell membrane as the 'doorman', for it governs all movement in and out of the cell. Changes in the level of hydration within the body mean changes in the communication between cells. If you imagine the full spectrum of light moving through a distorted, gross cell membrane, the light would be refracted and come out of the other side of the cell with part of its spectrum missing. This diminished message would then be passed on from cell to cell. When we become dehydrated, the cell membrane also loses its ability to hold and store photons and our worldview is literally darkened.

Maintaining the correct pH balance within the body is also vital for wellbeing. Many of the enzymes within our digestive system are switched on and off by changes in pH within the digestive tract. If we become too acidic, we literally lose the ability to digest our food correctly because the enzymes needed to do this work cannot be activated. We are actually slightly alkaline beings, but all aspects of our metabolism produce some acidity every day, so we have to rectify this by the end of each 24-hour cycle in order to return to our natural condition. An inability to achieve this is reflected in our whole being and we see this situation in people who have acid thoughts and display acidic behaviour. Headaches and achiness are other indications that the pH balance is not correct. When we are too acidic, our worldview again becomes darker and more contracted, and this in turn robs us of the ability to see how to navigate through life effectively and to achieve real quality of life.

Temperature is also very important to our balance and wellbeing and it would appear as if many more people nowadays are becoming physically and emotionally colder and more cut off than in the past. When I was training for nursing some 40 years ago I was taught about body temperature and what was considered the average temperature for a human being. In looking at more recent nursing textbooks, I see that the figure given today is actually one degree lower than it was when I was first training and I can find no explanation for this in the medical literature. When we look at the role of iodine and the thyroid in the maintenance of the correct body temperature, however, it will become obvious why this is the case.

Minerals play a vital role in all aspects of human biochemistry and a lack of certain minerals can have a dramatic effect on health. In the west of Scotland, for example, intensive farming has depleted the soil of magnesium. Magnesium, sometimes called the 'great soother', is important for our inner sense of wellbeing. When we are deficient in it we tend to seek other, often synthetic chemicals to make us feel better. It is also vital for correct heart function. What we find in the west of Scotland is a very high consumption of sugar, high levels of alcoholism and drug addiction and very high levels of heart disease. These situations are all connected, but this is not currently acknowledged or even considered. We will also see that a lack of magnesium can dramatically reduce our ability to cleanse and rebalance at a cellular level.

Getting the mineral balance correct in our vehicle is vital for health. Too much or too little of the minerals required can cause disharmony and sometimes have long-term implications.

Many minerals work in tandem and are energetically opposed to each other. Two that work in this way are zinc and copper. When a baby is in utero, the mother's body has to prepare to give birth to it. This is a process of separating off in order to make the baby less dependent. Within the uterus the baby is totally dependent upon its mother. Part of our purpose as humans is to achieve independent thought so that our uniqueness can be fully expressed. An important aspect of growing up is achieving more independence. So, towards the end of her pregnancy, a mother's copper levels will rise, causing a recessive influence upon zinc. The effect of copper is quite convulsive and is an important part of the mechanisms of the contraction of labour. Once the baby is born, the mother's copper levels should naturally reduce and her zinc levels should rise. Eating the placenta raises zinc levels (humans are the only mammals who do not eat their own placenta). If the mother's zinc levels do not rise, the child can become very dependent, and if this situation continues beyond puberty, the dependence can continue well into adulthood. We know that the contraceptive pill is very high in copper and when you consider that it is common to prescribe this early in puberty to ease menstrual pain, you can see what a potentially detrimental effect this can have.

The transitions we make in life are so crucial to our ability to fulfil our true potential. Birth and puberty are important transitions that need to be navigated with both care and wisdom. The transitions into motherhood and the menopause are equally important. Each transition brings with it the potential for a dramatic change in consciousness. If the vehicle is supported correctly through each of the transitions, the potential of the individual grows and expands. If, however, any kind of stress or suppression occurs around the time of a transition, it can have dramatic consequences.

One of the most striking connections I have made in my 35 years of working with people is the fact that in 90 per cent of the patients I have treated with anorexia, the condition arose within six months of having the BCG vaccination during their teens. All vaccinations give the body the resonance of a disease and the BCG vaccine gives the resonance of tuberculosis. Often, rather than guarding the individual against catching this disease, the BCG vaccine ignites dormant imbalances that have been carried forward from ancestors whose bodies had or carried TB. We are each born with predispositions that come from our ancestral line and these again need to be considered when understanding our own uniqueness.

In the West it is common to give children up to 32 different vaccines before the age of two. Giving a child who is going through an important transition from baby to toddler, with its many developmental milestones, the resonance of 32 different infections cannot be good sense.

Fear is a powerful tool when it comes to the world of vaccinations. When you consider that the continual increase in childhood problems such as autism and ADHD correlates so well with the increase in vaccination levels, you have to ask if conventional thinking on the fundamentals of health is in any way sound.

Collective Thought Can Change Belief Systems

The power of collective thought is huge in our society. Just think about the vast number of people who believe almost everything they are told by the media. There is a belief that certain things are incurable and unchangeable and that we have to make do and accept situations we do not like. However, a belief is just a thought that you have over and over again. If you change the way you think, you naturally change your beliefs, and what in one belief system might seem impossible, in another becomes a matter of course.

Nature provides us with all the tools we need in order to find balance and harmony. All we have to do is pick up those tools and use them. If you want to find balance, if you want to be healthy, you must take full responsibility for achieving it for yourself and by yourself. This is the only way to find health *and* freedom.

We think in the West that we are free, but for many people freedom is an illusion. Someone who is truly free can go anywhere in the world and be at peace with whatever they encounter. Our co-dependent natures prevent us from being able to do this. When most people plan holidays or go travelling, they would not consider visiting a place where they were not certain that they could get food, drink, money, the medicines they required and easy access to a doctor in case anything went wrong. This kind of approach makes the world a much more contracted place for us and places vast areas of this beautiful planet of ours out of bounds to us. The human being living in all the brilliance of their full potential does not have such restrictions. They understand that through thought alone they can attract anything that they might need anywhere on the planet.

How you think and what you think have the strongest influence upon your reality and this is especially true when it comes to your body. Some people do not like their body, some are frustrated or disappointed with the way it functions or apparently malfunctions, and others do not give it a second thought. Many people suffer from chronic conditions and are unable to bring about lasting change because they are forever focusing on their symptoms. This is like endlessly looking at a problem rather than actively seeking a solution.

Your body is amazing. It has incredible powers of resilience and healing, but it is the *mind* that is the master of it all. When the mind truly connects with the body it is like a light going on in every cell. The body becomes vibrant and connected and able to dance with universal rhythms. When this happens, with each passing day it heads steadily closer to balance and harmony.

So let me invite you to take a journey in your vehicle, a journey back to yourself. You require no special skills to make this journey successfully, just an open and enquiring mind. It is my intent that as you embark on this journey you start to make more and more connections. It is a bit like joining the dots to make a picture. And the more connections you make, the clearer you will be about who you really are.

I will share with you the founding principles on which my work is based. These principles are very simple but extraordinarily powerful. They form the foundation upon which we will build health and vitality.

I also want to show you how the body really works in a way that is easily understandable. Once you have this understanding you will be able to see much more clearly how and why the body appears to malfunction.

We will also explore the true nature and purpose of disease. You will learn exactly how and why disease arises and how to release it from the body. I will show you how modern medicine is actually based upon an inaccurate theory and how it is through a lack of understanding of the true nature of disease that chronic illness arises.

Once we have made these connections, it becomes possible to understand the process of bringing the body back to harmony and full potential. This is achieved through three stages of treatment, which are once again simple and easily understandable. Over the past 35 years of practice I have acquired a broad range of techniques that can be used to support the body on its journey back to health. These techniques are hugely empowering because they provide you with tools to bring about change in a very short space of time. If the body becomes in any way overburdened with toxicity, it has an immediate effect on how we function, feel and think. Techniques help to create movement and space, enabling us to ease the burden on the body and to free the mind. Each technique is simple and easy to do with the minimum of equipment.

One of the most important aspects of my work with patients is taking the case history, because it is through this that one begins to understand a patient's story. By looking at the patient's life and also the health of parents and grandparents, we can begin to see the journey that has been undertaken to bring the person to the place where they currently find themselves. Interpreting the case history is often a revelatory experience for patients, as it is the time when there is a great joining of the dots and in doing so they begin to understand their own story and what it means. I will share with you some case histories to show this process in action and these will greatly assist you in understanding your own story.

Once you understand your own story, you can then begin to write a new story for yourself – a story of health, happiness and freedom. It can be an adventure story where the hero or heroine overcomes every adversity, masters all problems and lives happily ever after. It can be whatever story you want it to be. When you write your own story, even apparently insurmountable odds can be overcome. Miracles become possible, hope is restored and passion ignited. You truly take charge of your own reality.

So let our journey begin.

CHAPTER 2

WATER: THE LIQUID CRYSTAL FROM ABOVE TO BELOW

Let us begin our journey by looking at how we record the messages of the universe within our bodies.

Our bodies are made up of 70 per cent water and the ratio of solid matter to water within them is the same as the ratio of land to ocean on planet Earth. Water is life and without it no creature or plant could survive. It is the cradle that holds the universal messages in and around every living cell of every living thing on the Earth. We are going to see that if this vital fluid component of our body becomes contracted, our ability to hold the positive energies of our universe becomes contracted too.

We refer to water as 'the liquid crystal from above to below'. This means that it holds universal wisdom and transports it from the macrocosm to the microcosm, right into the cell. It is so fundamental to life that our body has a built-in protective process that it takes on as soon as it feels dehydrated. Contrary to what we might have been told, the body *never* works against us. It always does the very best it can for us given the circumstances we present it with.

People living in arid countries also have ways to maintain hydration within their culture. For example, in Morocco the women working in the fields don't take a lot of water with them; instead they take freshly pressed argon oil. We see how certain cultures have retained the knowledge that a very important ingredient for maintaining hydration is oil containing essential fatty acids. More on these later.

So what causes us to become dehydrated in the first place? Our first principle, indeed the founding principle of cellular awakening, is that any kind of stress is registered on the water component of the body as dehydration. Furthermore, as soon as the body is dehydrated, it is expressed as stress. So external stress causes cellular dehydration, which then causes internal stress. This creates a Catch-22 situation within the body, because internal stress will be registered on the water component of the body as further dehydration.

When you consider that a fully functioning brain is 80 per cent water, it is easy to see that the brain is one of the first places to register dehydration. It has been found that in some cases of very deep depression, the brain can be dehydrated to as much as 40 per cent of its normal capacity. This creates a person who is very cut off from their full potential and the full experience of universal wisdom.

In the five element theory of Chinese medicine, it is understood that fear and stress are held within the element of Water. This element controls and sustains the kidneys, brain and central nervous system. This perspective is not so different from the Western perspective, because we know that the kidneys control fluid levels in the body and that the brain has the highest proportion of water of any organ in the body. Traditional Chinese doctors know that all thoughts are vibrations and that if the resonance of any kind of stress, whether it's a job you do not like or an unresolved emotion, is held within the body for two years, then there is always a manifestation within the water component as dehydration. This means that if there is anything in your life that you are unhappy about, it will, if left unresolved for two years, create a contraction of your ability to be in tune with the universe.

Dr Masaru Emoto's Experiments with Water

Some amazing experiments have been undertaken recently that have vividly illustrated water's ability to hold messages. Perhaps the most spectacular were those carried out by Dr Masaru Emoto. Dr Emoto, a Japanese scientist, became interested in finding a simple way to test the purity and energetic vitality of water. It had long been known that certain natural waters had healing properties, but science had never been able to substantiate this. After seeing pictures of snowflakes, Dr Emoto wondered if water could be frozen in such a way as to reveal its crystalline structure. After many months he perfected a process that froze distilled water into a crystalline form. He photographed this frozen water to reveal the beauty of the crystal structures.

Next he wondered if the nature of water could be changed by subjecting it to different vibrations. To test his theory he took two glass bottles of distilled water from the same source and subjected them to two different messages. On separate pieces of paper he wrote, in Japanese, the words 'love' and 'hate' and he taped one word to each bottle so that the letters were facing inwards. He then left these bottles overnight and the next day froze and photographed the water. The water from the bottle labelled with 'love' produced crystals of extraordinary beauty. However, the water from the bottle labelled with 'hate' produced deformed and chaotic crystals. From this he began to understand that water had the ability to hold vibrations, and went on to conduct many hundreds of experiments subjecting distilled water to different words, music and other vibrational influences. On each occasion he found that vibrations that felt good produced beautiful crystals and vibrations that felt uncomfortable produced distorted crystals.

Having proven his theory that water was influenced by different vibrations, he wondered if the water component of food might be equally influenced. He chose a simple food with a high water content, namely cooked short-grain brown rice (which, interestingly, is 70 per cent water, the same as the human body). In Chinese medicine short-grain brown rice is known as 'the food of the colon', which is the organ that holds the message of whether we are dehydrated or not. Dr Emoto decided to take cooked brown rice and divide it into three glass jars. The first one he left aside as the control. The second one he hurled abuse and negative thoughts at whenever he could. The third one he loved, nurtured and sent extremely positive thoughts to. He did this every day for a period of 10 days. When he then looked at the short-grain brown rice in the jars he found something very interesting. The rice in the control jar had naturally fermented to a degree where you would not want to eat it. The abused rice was dry, dark and hard and in no way edible. The rice that had been nurtured had fermented but was still sweet enough to eat. We can see clearly how the water held within the rice was receiving the messages and vibrations and recording them. It is not only what you eat that affects your health, but the thoughts and feelings you hold while you are preparing and eating that food.

A Hydrated Body and the Four Electrolytes

To better understand how the body operates when fully hydrated, we can look at the movement of our four main electrolytes, sodium, potassium, calcium and magnesium. These electrolytes actually charge the body by charging the water and depending upon the charge they are holding they can move water in and around the body. In a fully hydrated person this means having the ability to freely move messages around the body.

Sodium and calcium always partner together and their natural position is outside the cell in what is called the 'extracellular fluid'. However, during the daytime, when the sun is dominant over the moon, we are in active mode and it is light, a significant amount of that sodium and calcium pass through the cell membrane and into the cell. The sodium, as it moves into the cell, will displace potassium, and the calcium, as it moves in, will displace magnesium.

During the hours of darkness this whole process is reversed. The moon has a great affinity for sodium, as we see with the tides, and so at night, when activity diminishes, the moon is dominant and it is dark, the sodium and calcium are drawn back out through the cell membrane and at the same time the magnesium and potassium move back into the cell. When this process is complete, you have the perfect exchange of electrolytes. The build-up of sodium and calcium inside the cell is part of feeling tired. In order to restore balance we need to lie prone, rest and sleep. This is perfect because it enables so many rebalancing processes to take place within us.

In a fully hydrated person this also represents the perfect polarity, because in this pushing out to return the body to normal, you have two potassiums coming in to push out three sodiums, meaning there is more positive charge going out than coming back in. This happens in order to maintain a correct charge inside and outside the cell, because if you have only two positive ions coming in with three going out, the inside of the cell membrane will be more negative and the outside of the cell membrane will maintain a more positive charge. Then negatively charged particles will congregate in clusters around the cell membrane, forming what are called 'electron clouds'. These electron clouds accept the photons of light; they hold light. When this happens we have the macrocosm, universal wisdom, being held outside the cell membrane of each and every one of the trillions of cells in the body. Messages from the macrocosm are then transported, via water, through the cell membrane into the microcosm.

So, when the cell membrane holds the correct charge and polarity, we can access universal wisdom, live our lives to the full and realize our potential for expression and expansion. The cell membrane potential is intrinsically linked to the life potential.

We live in an ever-changing universe and in order for us to be able to dance to the universal rhythms, we need to have a complete transfer of universal wisdom into our cells on a daily basis. Complete transfer can only occur in someone who is fully hydrated and thus holding the correct charge. This requires that by the end of each night all of the sodium and calcium has left the inside of the cell and returned to its normal place outside the cell. So the day/ night cycle is the first of the universal rhythms to which we must dance if we are to flow with all that is around us.

Dehydration Alert

Let us now look at what happens at a cellular level within a dehydrated body. We have said that the body never works against us. It always, without exception, does the very best it can for us at any given point in time. When we are dehydrated it will protect us, but if we don't address that dehydration, we become arrested at that point in time. It is one of the body's defence mechanisms. But this creates a situation where we tend to live in the past rather than the present.

So how does the body respond when it first registers dehydration? It immediately goes into a state of heightened alertness that we refer to as 'dehydration alert'. Through the action of the liver, it then increases the production of cholesterol, which is transported to the dehydrated cells.

The cell membrane is a triple layer. There are two polarization layers on the outer sides that hold the charge that we have just been talking about, and in the centre there is a lipid layer, which carries no charge. When the body produces this extra cholesterol, it places it within the cell membrane to protect against further water loss. This reduces the permeability of the cell membrane, which in turn affects the ability of the channels within the cell membrane to open and close. This reduced permeability interferes with the normal movement of the four electrolytes into and out of the cell.

This interference can have a marked effect on our health, but it is a natural reaction to a given situation. It is the body working to protect us from serious harm. The function of the cholesterol is to protect the fluid inside the cell so that we don't dehydrate to death.

During the day, the force of the sun is strong enough to power the movement of the sodium and calcium into the cell, displacing the potassium and magnesium. However, the effect of the moon on us is much gentler. This creates a situation where at night the power of the moon to draw the sodium and calcium back out through the triple-layered cell membrane that is coated with cholesterol is diminished. What we also find, especially in the Western diet, is that we are deficient in magnesium, and magnesium is required to enable its partner potassium to move back

THE DAY/NIGHT CYCLE (IN A HYDRATED BODY)
A normal healthy cell – electrolyte movement by DAY

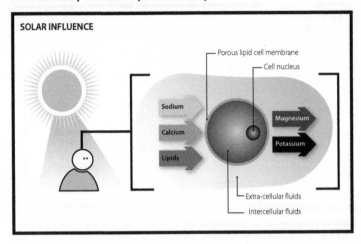

The natural position for **Na** and **Ca** is outside the cell. The natural position for **Mg** and **K** is inside the cell. Daytime – the sun pushes the Na/Ca + lipids (which always travel together) into the cell. This displaces their opposites – Na displaces K, Ca displaces Mg. The lipid cell membrane is porous due to adequate EFA in the diet.

A normal healthy cell – electrolyte movement by NIGHT

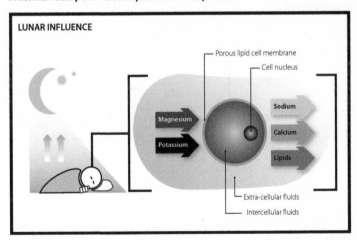

Night-time – The moon draws the **Na** (bringing the **Ca** and lipids with it as they always travel together) out of the cell. This is aided by a push from the **Mg** and **K** in their return to the inside of the cell. The lipid cell membrane is porous due to adequate EFA in the diet.

THE DAY/NIGHT CYCLE (IN A DEHYDRATED BODY)
A dehydrated cell – electrolyte movement by **DAY**

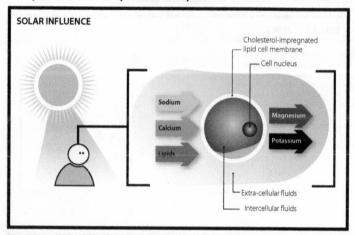

Here the cell membrane is far less porous than it should be – creating resistance to the electrolyte movement. However, during the day the energy push by the sun is strong, so the **Na, Ca** and lipids are not too inhibited by the cholestrol coating and so are able to push their way in, displacing the **Mg** and **K**.

A dehydrated cell – electrolyte movement by **NIGHT**

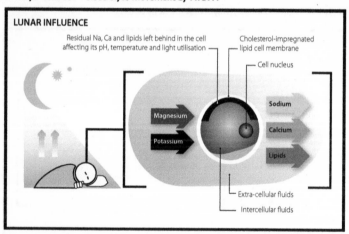

Here the cell membrane is far less porous than it should be, creating resistance to the electrolyte movement. As the moon pull is far gentler than the sun push, the night-time exchange of the electrolytes is more impeded. In addition the Western diet is high in **Na/Ca** but short in **Mg/K**, so the **Mg/K** levels required to carry out the push back into the cell are not present. All of the above results in a residue of **Na, Ca** and lipids being left behind in the cell.

into the cell at night. So during the daytime we have the movement of sodium in, but during the night-time the cell does not manage to move all of the sodium out again. The incomplete movement means that we have more sodium, with its positive charge, within the cell than we should have, and so the conditions inside the cell start to change.

The charge inside the cell is the first thing to change. This means that our stresses manifest inside our cells and the immediate effect is that the cell membrane potential is diminished and we lose the ability to hold electron clouds. So we immediately lose the ability to hold all the messages coming to us, via light, from the universe. We are not receiving what is rightfully ours and not responding in the way that we normally would. We have stopped dancing correctly to the rhythm of the day/night exchange. We are not in tune. This causes a lack of ease that is the first manifestation of the dis-ease process.

I see this situation very clearly in someone who is manifesting ME (myalgic encephalopathy, or chronic fatigue syndrome). I will ask them, 'What do you feel like after a night's sleep?' and they will often say that they actually feel worse than before they went to bed. The build-up of positive charge within the cell needs to be dispersed during the night, it needs to be lost from inside the cell for that person to not have any manifestation of dis-ease. The answer here lies in helping the person to rehydrate. Just taking a medicine or remedy will potentially add more stress to the body because it is another message that has to be deciphered. And if you take a homoeopathic remedy, it can only fulfil its potential to the levels of your hydration.

When the charge inside the cell is not correct, it also means that the pH level in the cell is not correct. And if the pH in the cell is not right, the pH in the whole body will be wrong. Remember when we talked about the body as a test tube we said that hydration, pH, temperature and ability to hold and utilize light were all important factors. Looking at somebody who is on dehydration alert, we can see that the hydration has changed, the pH has changed, the light availability has changed, because we have this interference with the formation of electron clouds, and because it is closing down, the cell will also start to change temperature, becoming colder. The more dehydration is present, the colder a person becomes.

One of the things we see is that under these circumstances the person loses their ability to produce acute episodes of illness. The person with ME has lost the ability to have a beautifully flamboyant cold or 'flu manifestation where the body has the energy to warm itself up. So on dehydration alert we start to see stagnation and all of the illnesses that are connected with stagnation. If the lymph is stagnant, for example, we might see constant ear infections in children. Low energy is a strong sign of stagnation.

If the stagnation becomes extreme, it can affect brain function quite dramatically. Someone manifesting a schizoid episode, for example, is actually in a state of extreme dehydration. Hyperactivity, bi-polar disorder and strange behaviour all indicate a condition where a person is becoming more and more closed off from the universe. A person who it seems is living out a somewhat mad and bizarre existence, such as someone with extreme mental illness, is a person who is cut off from outer influences and whose entire being is going on within. This kind of person is locked into themselves, into an altered sense of reality that is in no way connected to universal wisdom. They think and behave without reference to what is really going on outside and find socializing all but impossible.

The deeper the level of dehydration, the deeper and more serious the disease. We can see that a situation such as cancer is going to have a very dehydrated picture and therefore a very fearful picture. When a person is very dry, there is a strong message of fear coming from within their own body.

What we find in these so-called 'incurable' diseases is that we have a Catch-22 situation where the stress and fear drive the dehydration, and the dehydration drives the fear and stress. There is no point in coming in here with an intellectual rationale as to why the person is ill and saying that because they are so ill they need to take masses of medications or remedies. What we need to do first is reassure the body by switching off the dehydration alert. We have to encourage the day/night cleanse rather than throw in a whole load of other things, because if we do that, the body is going to receive many more messages, which will create more stress, driving the body to produce more cholesterol that will further cut down the cellular exchange.

Perhaps we need to consider the possibility that we create degenerative disease by sending more and more messages to a body that can no longer hear who it is. A person cannot be driven towards true healing by being bombarded with external messages in the form of medications and remedies (orthodox or alternative). In cases of serious illnesses, such as cancer, you have a situation where the person has no connection to their inner wisdom. This explains why they are so often driven to take on board rather horrific treatments.

When the dehydration alert is present it also influences energy. Martin L. Budd, in his book *Low Blood Sugar*, describes hypoglycaemia (low blood sugar) as the inability to hold calcium levels correctly within the blood. We can see that if calcium is stuck along with sodium inside a cell, it is not possible to maintain stable blood sugar and this immediately impacts energy levels. So any situation that causes dehydration is also going to cause a drop in energy potential. This in turn has a very profound effect on every part of the body. This can lead to a wide variety of problems such as lymph congestion, high blood pressure, tiredness and a weakened immune system.

Fundamentally, what we are saying is that if there is any kind of disease present within the body, dehydration will naturally already be there. This is because when the cellular exchange does not take place, a person becomes gradually more and more toxic. All illness, be it fluid retention, headaches, constipation or extreme illness, takes us back to our first principle: the person must be dehydrated.

What Can Make Us Dehydrated?

So what sorts of things in our lives and environment cause us to be dehydrated? We have already said that anything that causes us stress or makes us fearful leads to dehydration. This can be in our relationships, in our job or in our home. It can be our journey to work, the places we frequent and all sorts of other things. Of course it can also be things from the past. Unresolved emotions are held within the body as vibrations ticking away in the background but drawing towards them similar vibrations from the macrocosm. This is how sometimes people seem to consistently attract the same kind of destructive situations in their lives over and over again. But when we open the cells to receive universal wisdom, we can revisit and release these old vibrations that are no longer relevant to our lives and release the blockages from the past that are stopping us from moving forward.

As well as stress from unresolved emotions, we also have environmental stresses placed upon us. The very worst of these is electromagnetic interference from things such as mobile phones and wi-fi. It can be very challenging, for instance, to live near to a mobile phone mast. We are endlessly bombarded with these hidden energies and they can have a huge impact on what is unfolding in and around our cell membranes. These kinds of energies can directly affect our cell membrane potential. In doing so they affect our sense of who we really are and, remember, the biggest stress of all is not knowing who we are and not manifesting it. Mobile and digital phones, computers, electric blankets and a lot of electrical equipment, especially in the bedroom, all create potentially harmful fields of electromagnetic interference.

The amount of flying that many people do these days further exposes the body to electromagnetic stress. Just think about sitting in an airport with all of the communication that is going on there. The air is literally teeming with electromagnetic interference.

When looking for causes of stress in a person's life we need to consider lifestyle, but we can also look at drugs, both prescribed and social, and we can look at diet. Consider the challenge of a commercially prepared hamburger and fries as opposed to a bowl of fresh homemade soup.

You can also see how putting too much sodium in your diet and not enough potassium can be potentially very stressful. We need to create a potassium dominance in what we choose to eat and drink if we are to achieve and maintain our full potential, both at a cell membrane and a human level. The Western diet tends to have a dominance of sodium and calcium.

Then we can look at how we treat illness. Most people who become ill these days seem to be obsessed with obliterating symptoms. That is a very suppressive process.

We can also look at vaccinations. Vaccinations, once given, remain in the body as the vibration of an illness which perhaps a person may meet at some time in their life. Do you not think that holding the vibration of a disease within you will attract similar vibrations to it? Today, as already mentioned, we see that there is the potential for a child to have had 32 vaccines, that is the vibrational message of 32 illnesses, by the time it is two years of age.

It is very easy to see how our society, which is totally and utterly fear driven, becomes more and more contracted and closed off from universal wisdom. And if we live in a body that is similarly closed off, just think how small our vision is and how easy we are to control.

So our work in this book is primarily to switch off the dehydration alert, because we know that if a cell remains coated in cholesterol, it is not going to allow us to recreate the perfect day/night movement of the sodium and calcium and the potassium and magnesium.

How to Switch Off the Dehydration Alert System

To biochemically switch off the body's dehydration alert is quite a lengthy process. We need to change the structure of the cell membrane in order to be able to fully hydrate and utilize light, and this takes time. However, earlier on I mentioned that the colon is the organ that registers whether the body is hydrated or not, and it is within this organ that we can mechanically turn off the dehydration alert within the body.

It is not possible to have an allergy, for example, unless you produce histamines. The cells that produce histamines are the mast cells, a majority of which are found in the colon. It is not possible for the mast cells in your colon to produce histamine unless you are dehydrated. So our point of focus is going to be our diet and lifestyle and how those are registered in our colon.

Look at your own lifestyle. How often do you use a mobile phone? How often have you got it turned on? Do you have an 'old-fashioned' wired telephone at home or do you now use a cordless phone? Perhaps it might be better for you to have a wired phone. How often do you use your computer? Do you have a television in your bedroom? Do you turn electrical equipment off or is it forever on standby? Do you have an electric blanket? Do you use a microwave? Do you travel every day of the week on the electrified subway or train? Think how all these things might be affecting your polarity.

It is essential to address all areas of stress, because if we do not turn off the body's dehydration alert, we have no way of naturally helping it to achieve the correct cellular exchange. Anything else will be just working against it and causing more stress.

Are you helping your body stay in balance by trying to work with the natural rhythms of the environment? In the northern hemisphere we have a shortened light span during the winter, making the nights longer. This is no accident of nature. In the winter we have an increase in our metabolisms that takes place in order for us to maintain body warmth and so need the longer nights to give our cells more time to cleanse and rebalance. If we have 14 hours of darkness, we should ideally be resting during those 14 hours because that is the time it will take for our day/night exchange to fully unfold. In the summer, when there is a lot more light, you don't need as long. So if you have the opportunity to tailor your lifestyle to be more in tune with the light and the dark, I would suggest that you take it.

Having looked briefly at lifestyle, let us now consider how diet can help to switch off the dehydration alert registered in our colons. Our diet needs to be hydrating and reassuring to the colon. Simple eating helps to remove stress and allows the body to have spare energy and therefore the spare potential to heal. A simple, natural diet contains simple messages that can quickly bring the body back into balance.

We need to eat foods that help to balance the pH, that are not going to challenge our blood sugar. For instance, if we are considering grains, we need to make sure that we choose ones that do not over-challenge insulin production.

It is also not natural for us to eat after dark, as this is the natural time for rest and rejuvenation. Digestion takes huge amounts of energy over several hours after eating and so eating after dark can cause added stress to the body. In the winter most people do not arrive home from work until after dark, so it might be preferable to prepare only a simple meal at this time. Perhaps you might even choose to have a mono-meal such as a bowl of brown rice or a soup made with only one or two vegetables, so that you are not putting stress on the body to interfere with the more reflective time of winter. In the summer you can do the opposite and have a much more expanded menu.

Once we have mechanically turned off the dehydration alert in a patient it actually helps the person to get more in touch with themselves. If you are supporting hydration, you are also supporting the central nervous system, so the brain and mind become clearer. We are then ready to move on and change the biochemistry. We use diet and techniques to gradually change the conditions in the test tube so that the cellular cleanse becomes perfect. Techniques are my favourite aspect of cellular awakening. They are simple yet powerful tools that can give energy back to areas of the body that are very deprived of it. This creates increased movement and hydration, which in turn supports the central nervous system. This makes techniques potentially hugely consciousness altering.

To increase cell membrane permeability we also need to gradually improve the ability of the body to utilize oils, because the lipid cell membrane needs essential fatty acids to function correctly. How we do this will be explained on page 46.

*****

So, to recap, we are saying that the water component of our body holds the message of who we are but also holds our charge, and the polarity created by this charge is basically how we manifest who we are. If we work to change our polarity we must not be surprised to find that we also invite in a whole different kind of life. We create a new reality. When the charge of the cell membrane is correct, with the positive outside and negative inside, we can attract the electrons which in turn attract the photons in which is held the wisdom of the universe. In cellular awakening we work as facilitators helping people to open up and expand their potential so that they reacquire the ability to create their own reality and expand their being.

We have incredible bodies which are always seeking to find balance and harmony. If we just take the time to give some attention to our magnificent selves, we will discover the amazing potential held within our vehicle. Once someone has the ability to hold their own electron clouds around their cell membranes, they are in touch with all the information they need to move into a state of health and vitality.

If adequate photons (light) and oxygen are present in the body then the transmutation of electrolytes can take place. For example sodium into potassium. It is known that there are not enough channels in the cell membranes to allow all the exchange of electrolytes needed during the 24-hour cycle to be physical movement, so transmutation would account for the rest.

CHAPTER 3

LIGHT: OUR THREAD OF CONNECTION

Everything that we hear, see and experience in our universe is connected, and light is the connecting thread. In this chapter I will explain how our body utilizes light in the way that we communicate and how we pick up information, via light, from everyone we meet. Some people have a particular talent for picking up a sense of other people just by being with them. We call this empathizing. But it is in fact very difficult for anyone to really cover up who they are.

Because we are on the subject of light, I will also be talking about the two essential fatty acids. Essential fatty acids are so called because the body cannot make them itself but must obtain them from the diet. The two fatty acids that are essential to each and every one of us are omega 3 and omega 6. These two substances have an amazing potential to work with light.

The Disconnection between Eastern and Western Medicine

In the modern world of medicine and healing, East and West have become separated, yet everything *is* connected. In the East, for instance, it is quite normal to talk about chakras. Chakras are the light and energy centres of the body and each chakra is expressed as a different colour. What is not so well understood is that behind each of the chakras is one of our endocrine glands. Here we can see East and West making a connection.

In order to be healthy we have to understand what is needed to service the endocrine glands. They have a very important role to play in utilizing light, being connected to both the light coming into us and the light coming out of us. It is not widely known that each of us not only utilizes light in our bodies but also produces and emits it too, but today it can be shown scientifically that each cell of our body has the potential to create light. Experiments have shown that when a positive free radical and a negative free radical come together in the body, the force of their collision is such that a photon of light is produced.

Light coming from the macrocosm into our bodies enters through the chakras and it is now believed that it travels all around our bodies on the acupuncture meridians. Again, in the East there is an understanding of the acupuncture meridians that move *chi* (energy) around our bodies. Each acupuncture meridian has a relationship with different organs and different emotions. Along each meridian there are acupuncture points which relate to the outer universe as well as our inner universe. The light coming in from outside enters our bodies and moves along the meridians.

There has also been a great deal of talk of late about our 'light body'. The light body exists within the physical body. These are all ancient pieces of information that have become disconnected from one another.

In the last chapter we talked about the dehydrated cell. We discussed how when the body goes on dehydration alert it changes the structure of the cell membrane in such a way that the movement of light in and out of the cell becomes more and more impaired.

The Aborigines say that the way our body communicates is with light, but they also say that our cells communicate with one another via colour. Within light there are all of the colours of the spectrum, from violet to red. Let us imagine the full spectrum of light coming towards a fully functioning cell. It enters it and then leaves it and moves on to another cell, and to another and so on. If, however, the cell is dehydrated, then the light entering it will be refracted and only part of the full spectrum will emerge out of the other side. This means that a different message will be passed through that cell to the next one. Dehydration alert affects the penetration of light and essential nutrients through the cell membrane and thus the quality of communication we receive.

It is our responsibility to ensure that the conditions in our test tube are correct for the utilization of everything coming into our cells. Perhaps the most difficult thing to utilize is oil. I frequently have patients who come to me with a really deep understanding that oil is important but who display very strange symptoms when they start to take it. When this happens we need to look at the conditions in the test tube. We look at hydration and if necessary switch off the dehydration alert. We also look at the availability of light and light utilization, the pH and the temperature. To correct the pH, we use an alkalizing diet alongside techniques. Remembering that the endocrine system uses light, we also look at how impaired that system is. The thyroid, one of the endocrine glands, is very important in the control of body temperature. We know that if a person has a lowered body temperature, then the functioning of the thyroid will most probably be impaired. Changes in body temperature affect the endocrine system, which in turn affects our utilization of oils and therefore light and our ability to create light. We must not forget that the macrocosm is represented in the light that we receive and that the important thing is to allow the maximum amount of the macrocosm to get inside our cells and thus into our microcosm, so that we can match our environment as closely as possible.

The Cell's Charge and Electron Clouds

Let us now look a little more closely at the cell. The cell needs to hold the correct electrical charge. This is because when we take the essential fatty acids into our body, that is omega 3 and omega 6, they have the potential to create a lot of electron clouds, and electrons have the ability to accept the photons of light which hold the message of the universe.

When the conditions in the test tube are correct, the essential fatty acids are quickly and efficiently broken down and metabolized and produce electron clouds. These clouds are composed of negatively charged subatomic particles. In order to be able to attract them to the outside of the cell membrane, the charge on the outside of the cell membrane must become very positive by the end of each 24-hour cycle. The clouds need to be held around the cell membrane, because if they float off they will not have the correct effect and the messages that are delivered via the photons will not enter the cell.

So, in order to get in touch with our own wisdom, we need to be working on the nutritional requirements within the cell. We need the nucleus to have a strong positive charge, the inside of the cell membrane to have a strong negative charge and the outside of the cell membrane to have a strong positive charge. This enables the negatively charged electrons to be held around the outside of the cell membrane. This is why the cell membrane potential is so crucially important. There also needs to be a substantial difference between the charge inside and outside the cell.

The overall charge of the cell changes depending upon where in the 24-hour cycle we are and is very dependent upon our state of health. It takes a full 24-hour cycle to return the cell to its correct charge in a healthy individual. The Earth also changes its charge over the course of each 24 hours.

Regarding electron clouds, the more evolved a person or animal is, the more electron clouds are found accumulating outside the cell membrane, and the easier it is for the person or animal not only to pick up all of the information coming into them but also to emit correctly who they are. To put it simply, the larger the electron clouds, the more light a person carries and radiates.

Interestingly, only whales, dolphins and humans have the ability to create chains containing 28 carbon atoms, while all other animals create chains of 26 carbon atoms. The longer these chains, the greater their ability to hold light and thus the greater the level of potential enlightenment.

Omega 3 and Omega 6

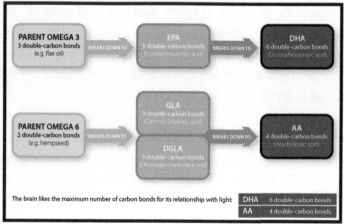

THE BREAKDOWN OF OMEGA 3 AND 6

Omega 3 and omega 6 are the only essential fatty acids for humans. Some people think that omega 9 is also essential, but in fact the body can produce omega 9 from omega 3, so it isn't essential. So what is it that is so special about these two fatty acids, particularly in relation to light and the endocrine system?

Omega 3 and omega 6 are required to produce substances called *prostaglandins*, which serve the endocrine system. For our bodies to be able to produce the full range of required prostaglandins we need omega 3, omega 6, magnesium, zinc and the vitamins B3, B6, C and E. These substances need to be available continuously for prostaglandins to be produced and thus the endocrine system to function at its full potential.

So where is the connection with light? Let us look first at omega 3. An omega 3 oil, such as flax oil, has three double-carbon bonds. Our bodies break this down into EPA, which has five double-carbon bonds. The EPA is further broken down to DHA, which has six double-carbon bonds. The more broken down the oil is, the more double-carbon bonds it has. Omega 6 only has two double-carbon bonds. When that is broken down to GLA, it has three double-carbon bonds. This is further broken down into Arachidonic acid, which has four double-carbon bonds. So when we break down omega 3 we end up with DHA, which has six double-carbon bonds, and when we break down omega 6 we end up with four.

What is so beautiful is that the brain has a great requirement for DHA and Arachidonic acid, both of which have the largest potential to hold light. So the higher aspect of each of us, the brain, has much more potential to hold light than other parts of the body. DHA and Arachidonic acid do exist elsewhere in the body, but the greatest concentration is in the brain. However, if the conditions within the test tube are not correct, the person is unlikely to be able to break the essential oils down.

The Matching of Oils to the Geography of the Planet

Nature is amazing when you look at the different availability of oils in the world. If we look in the coldest, darkest area, the Arctic, we think of the Eskimos. What kind of oils are these people going to be consuming? What we find is that they are having fish oils, which are rich in EPA and DHA. These are oils with more double-carbon bonds and therefore more potential to hold light, which of course is needed when living in a dark climate.

If we move a little further south we find that flax oil is consumed, which is an omega 3 oil. Canada would be a good example and this is where a great deal of flax is grown. Interestingly, if you take flax to somewhere hotter and lighter, such as Brazil, and grow it there, it will grow very quickly, but it will not contain any omega 3. In any given environment nature will only produce food that is balanced for that environment.

Moving further south again into warmer and lighter conditions, we find that omega 6 starts to show up. Omega 6-rich oils include hemp, sunflower and pumpkin and have a higher level of omega 6 than of omega 3.

Then we move further south, for example to the Mediterranean, where there is yet more light and warmth. Here they use omega 9. Omega 9 is a mono-unsaturated fatty acid, meaning that is has just one double-carbon bond. The people living here have so much light available that they only need one carbon double-bond in their oils.

Moving even further south, to the equator, where there is a high level of strong sunlight, we find that the oils are saturated. Saturated oils have no double-carbon bonds, are very stable in heat and are also very important in the cell membrane, because saturated fats are better at creating structure than the unsaturated fats.

I have treated people manifesting a condition such as MS, who, when they are living in England, a fairly cold and dark country, need to use flax oil. But if they go and live, for example, in India for a period of time they actually find that they don't need to use that oil because they have moved into a hotter and lighter environment. I also frequently find with conditions such as ME, where people are clearly having difficulty utilizing light and where everything in their bodies is running slowly and is in a congested state, if you move them into a warmer, high-light environment, then the body starts to be able to pick up and communicate.

You can take this information about the planet regarding light, temperature and oils and transfer it into the body, into the test tube. So if the test tube is fairly cold and dark, you have to begin treatment by using the oils that are appropriate for colder and darker conditions.

In the very many books available on nutrition, you will find very different information on what is the correct ratio of omega 3 to omega 6 in our diets. There is a consensus of opinion that in a daily intake one would require more omega 6 than omega 3, but is this true and if so in what ratios? What we find is that different experts talk about different ratios. The more you explore the work of these individuals, the more you find that the ratio they recommend is dependent upon where in the world their research was undertaken. For example, if they carried out their research in a colder, darker place, they would find that a person would need a higher ratio of omega 3 to omega 6. I find in the British Isles that if I am working with someone living in Scotland in the winter, the requirement for omega 3 is going to be much higher than it will be during the summer. It is also interesting to note that when a cow is fed on good-quality green grass, the ratio of omega 3 to omega 6 is 1:1. However, if it is fed on grain, the ratio changes to 1:20 in favour of omega 6. The key lies in having your vehicle tuned into the conditions you are living in.

Dr Johanna Budwig and Light

Dr Johanna Budwig was one of the greatest researchers into how the body holds and utilizes light and was at the very forefront of understanding how light is crucial in the successful treatment of the very deep diseases such as cancer that are so prevalent today. She discovered just how important essential fatty acids were for holding knowledge and information and how their correct use could unlock our full potential as human beings. She also discovered that the sulphur-rich amino acids found in proteins needed to be taken at the same time as the essential fatty acids for the oils to be fully utilized. This is not surprising when you consider that in nature these oils always appear with protein, whether in a plant or animal. She understood that we need to be able to absorb these oils, move them through our lymphatic system and actually get them to the cell membrane.

In the very beginning of her treatments, Dr Budwig used to suggest that her patients did a flax-oil enema. She got them to insert 500ml of flax oil at body temperature into the anal cavity and to hold it there for one hour. She said that during that hour, that person would be receiving more electron-photon activity than they had ever received before. This would unlock their access to universal wisdom and enable them to find the answers to solve their own problems.

Oils are so important for hydration, and hydration is so important to stop fear. The work with Joanna Budwig and cancer is especially fascinating because she was actually saying that for a person to heal, they needed to have their internal antennae open to the full spectrum of light. Here she was not only talking about the colour spectrum, but also about ultraviolet and cosmic rays. She said that all of these rays held vital information that needed to be received into the physical body, held in the electron clouds and utilized by the cells. We know that if we are dehydrated and contracted, this is not possible because the charge around the cell membrane changes so that electron clouds do not form. We also know that if we are in this contracted state we are going to be fearful.

Remember we talked in the first chapter about the photon belt and how there was more photon availability in this current time than for the past 11,000 years? This means that more wisdom is available to us, but we can only access that wisdom if we have properly prepared our test tube. The increased light, lower magnetism and higher pulsing of the Earth all give us huge potential for change at a personal and global level. We began to enter the photon belt in 1987 and on 21 December 2012 we will be fully immersed, and we each need to make this transition.

Light not only comes in from the universe but is also produced by free radicals coming together at great speed. This internally-produced light is referred to as *bio-photons*. Our DNA personalizes the light from the universe. It holds the imprint of who we are, and when we are fully functioning and able to make and emit bio-photons, we are able to fully manifest who we are.

We can see how expressions such as *enlightenment* and being *all seeing* and *all knowing* are really talking about our ability to hold and utilize light. It is actually the light that is all seeing and all knowing. Within the light is the potential to see everything in a connected way, and that joyous connectedness means harmony, being at one with everything. This is not new knowledge but actually very ancient knowledge. The ancient Egyptian temples had special chambers where oils for anointing were mixed and other chambers designed specifically to facilitate the raising of the vibration of individuals. Anointing with oil is really anointing with light and has been linked to healing for many thousands of years, and healing is all about raising vibration and balancing energy.

When light and oxygen are present in sufficient quantities in the body, transmutation can take place. This completely changes the way we view our bodily functioning.

CHAPTER 4

THE UNIVERSAL CYCLES THAT WE DANCE TO

We are all individuals within this enormous universe. So how do we fit into the bigger picture and how does the bigger picture influence our body?

Every single thing around us has an influence upon us, because absolutely everything in our body, in our life and in the universe is connected. So let us look at some of the rhythms of nature to see how they influence us.

We will start with the day/night cycle that we discussed in Chapter 2. This is a cycle that involves the sun and the moon, both of which have profound influences upon us. Within that day/night cycle there are also two-hour periods where different organs, and therefore different emotions, are highlighted, as we shall see when we look at the Chinese five elements system in Chapter 6.

There are also shifts of energetic emphasis on different parts of our bodies as the moon moves through the different signs of the zodiac. These shifts occur every two to three days.

The monthly lunar cycle has an influence on all living things on this planet. Indeed, biodynamic gardeners are aware of this and are guided by the moon in their planting, pruning and harvesting. They know that there are completely different energies at work depending on whether the moon is expanding towards the full moon (called the *waxing moon*) or diminishing towards the new moon (called the *waning moon*).

Then we will see how the different seasons influence us. In Chinese medicine it is known that each of the seasons has a different influence upon our bodies. Each of our organs works cyclically with the unfolding seasons, and the different seasons have positive energetic influences upon different organs and emotions.

We will also look at the yearly cycle. Certain dates of the year, such as our birthday, can be potentially powerful times of change and rebalancing, but there are also nodal times that we can work with.

We will then take a journey beyond our planet to see how each of the planets in our solar system has an influence upon us.

Matching the Rhythms of Nature

To remain balanced, open and healthy, we each need to be able to dance with the rhythms of nature. The energies of nature ebb and flow during the day, month, season and year. When we dance with these energies our bodies cleanse and re-nourish on a daily basis. We can also take advantage of times of high energy to cleanse at a deeper level.

So let us remind ourselves how a healthy and hydrated body cleanses. When we talk about detoxifying, what we are talking about is the first cycle, the day/night cycle. During the daytime, when the sodium and calcium enter the cell and push out the potassium and magnesium, you have a change in the conditions within the cell. As the day progresses, the cell becomes more acidic, more toxic. The build-up of sodium and calcium and the diminution of potassium and magnesium are what leads to tiredness and the need to sleep. It is said that every hour we sleep before midnight is worth two hours of sleep after midnight, and in terms of our ability to effectively cleanse, this is correct.

Remember also that the oils we consume are very important in keeping the structure of the cell membrane permeable and thus healthy. At the end of the day, when we have a build-up of toxicity in our cells, it is natural to sleep and cleanse. During that time the sodium and calcium, under the attractive influence of the moon, move back out of the cell, and the potassium and magnesium move back in. As the sodium and calcium leave the cell, they bring with them toxicity. Once out of the cells, the toxins enter the lymphatic system. They move through it until they reach the blood. With each heartbeat, the lymph will drop into the blood. So the toxins move from the cell into the lymph and then into the blood. The blood flows around the body to the liver, which is the great filter. The liver extracts the toxicity from the blood, discharges it into the bile, and the bile flows via the common bile duct into the gall bladder. From here it travels into the duodenum, goes through the small intestines into the colon and finally out of the body. Toxins are also expelled through the skin and lungs. Every time we exhale we not only release carbon dioxide but also toxins. However, the movement from cell to lymph, lymph to blood, blood to liver, liver to bile and out is our primary route of detoxification. This route of elimination must be free flowing for us to remain healthy and we need to detoxify on a daily basis.

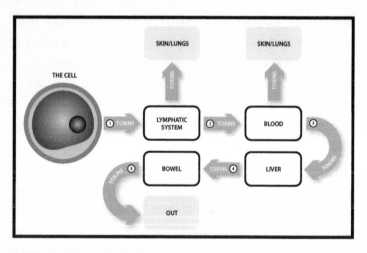

THE PRIMARY ROUTE OF ELIMINATION

If the night-time cleanse is complete and all of the sodium, calcium and toxicity leave the cell, the charge around the cell membrane will be correct by the end of the night. When this happens the person wakes up feeling refreshed, energized and ready for the day ahead. It is very common, however, for people to wake up tired in the morning even after a long night's sleep. This is because the cellular exchange of electrolytes is not fully functioning, therefore the person is not fully cleansing.

We can all feel the ebb and flow of the energies of the day/night cycle. Morning feels different from afternoon and afternoon feels different from evening. Our bodies dance with this ebb and flow, with the natural energies of the environment focusing on different parts of our bodies for a two-hour period each day.

The Day/Night Cycle

In the day/night cycle we see that the moon has a strong influence on sodium, but it also has further subtle influences on us. If you think of the zodiac as a means of marking the passage of time, the position of the moon in the zodiac changes roughly every two to three days. Each zodiac sign influences a different part of our body. So within the lunar month, as well as the drawing up and the letting go, every two to three days there is an emphasis upon a different part of our body as follows:

○ **The moon in Aries:** From the top of the head to the tip of the nose
○ **The moon in Taurus:** Jaws, neck and throat
○ **The moon in Gemini:** Shoulders, arms and hands

○ **The moon in Cancer:** From the lungs to the gall bladder
○ **The moon in Leo:** Heart and circulation
○ **The moon in Virgo:** Digestive organs
○ **The moon in Libra:** Hips, kidneys and bladder
○ **The moon in Scorpio:** Sexual organs
○ **The moon in Sagittarius:** Thighs
○ **The moon in Capricorn:** Knees, skin and bones
○ **The moon in Aquarius:** Lower leg
○ **The moon in Pisces:** Feet

The moon's influence further changes during its monthly cycle. During the waxing phase of the moon it is much easier for the cell to draw things into itself. During the waning phase of the moon it is much easier for the cell to release. This means that nurturing takes place more on the waxing moon and detoxifying more on the waning moon.

At the full moon there is a higher concentration of positive ions in the atmosphere. Most of us find concentrations of positive ions very uncomfortable. This is how we come to have the word 'lunatic', because the high level of positive ions around the time of the full moon has long been known to have a negative effect, especially on people with mental illness. Such people invariably have a very weak cell membrane potential and therefore find it too much of a struggle at a cellular level to adjust to these changes in the moon's charge.

Some people find it very useful to fast on the day of the full moon and indeed the body will find it most helpful to not have to use energy for digestion during this particular 24 hours. The high energy of the full moon gives the body a wonderful opportunity to cleanse at a deeper than normal level. However, the body must have enough spare energy to take advantage of this time. If nourishment was correct during the waxing moon, fasting for a day will be easy and very beneficial. The body must also be fully hydrated in order to be able to cleanse in this way.

At the new moon there are many more negative ions in the atmosphere, which for most of us is much more comfortable. That sense of inner ease makes the new moon another perfect time for the body to let go and detoxify, but in a much gentler way. Some people again choose to fast on the day of the new moon to allow the body as much energy as possible to cleanse, because at this time our potential for letting go is at its highest.

The Changing Influence of the Seasons

Let us look now at the influence of the changing seasons. Within the philosophy of Chinese medicine, each season is responsible for influencing different organs and each organ is linked to the expression of different emotions. So we have the two-hour periods of changing energy flow through different organs during the day, the two-day period influenced by the moon and now the seasonal periods, each of which lasts several weeks. This means there is a natural cycle in which each organ, and the emotion that organ expresses, is focused upon for a certain time in order to keep things moving in our bodies.

One of the classic signs of an inability to move with the seasonal rhythm is SAD (seasonal affective disorder). People with SAD tend to become affected in their minds and bodies when there is less light availability, such as during the winter. From the last chapter we know that anyone who suffers from SAD will have a poor essential fatty acid profile within their body.

Consuming the correct oils in the correct manner is vital if we are to be able to dance to the rhythm of the seasons, but correct overall nutrition is also essential. Rudolf Steiner said that if you keep feeding a child potatoes it will become locked into the mental level. This means that it will stop being able to move and express all of the different seasons within its body. With this it will be unable to express all the different emotions. An inability to express emotion has a marked effect on the mind and we become locked in our head. I see this situation in many adults and children with depression and mental illness. They have a constant internal dialogue unfolding in their minds that they cannot turn off. Fortunately, with the correct nutrition and support, the body and mind can always heal.

There are two special times of the year which Chinese physicians have always been very aware of. These are the spring equinox and the autumn equinox. The word 'equinox' means equal day and equal night, and the two equinoxes occur when the sun is at right angles to the equator. These are very specific energy times, the big changeovers between winter and summer.

At the spring equinox, usually around 21 March, we have equal hours of light and dark, after which we move into a time of gradually increasing hours of daylight. With each unfolding day there is more and more light available to us. This means an increase in photon activity. What happens on the spring equinox itself is that there is a sudden shift in our energy. During the winter our energy primarily moves up our back and down our front, but at the spring equinox this circulation flips and the energy then moves up our front and down our back, which has a much more expansive feel than the winter circulation.

The autumn equinox, around 21 September, also has equal hours of day and night, but after this the days get shorter and the nights get longer. There is therefore a reduction in the amount of photon activity with each passing day. On the autumn equinox our flow of energy again reverses and our energy once more moves up our back and down our front. This is a natural shift from the opening, expansive time of summer into the closing, introspective time of winter.

At the specific moments when this change takes place there is a huge surge of energy which detoxifies our cells. This means that we have two times of year when detoxifying is a natural event. This is why many people tend to get colds or 'flu around the times of the equinoxes.

We also have the solstices, which again are times of high energy, although there is no change in the flow of body energy at these times, so they don't have the same clearing and detoxifying influence. The summer solstice (in the northern hemisphere), around 21 June, is when the sun is directly over the Tropic of Cancer and is the longest day. The winter solstice, around 21 December, is when the sun is at right angles over the Tropic of Capricorn and is the longest night.

The influences of the sun and moon become even more amplified during solar and lunar eclipses and these represent further times of high energy.

The universe is forever moving and it asks us to move with it. If our cells are set up so that the day/night expression can fully unfold, every cell within our bodies will be fully charged and ready to dance with the two-hourly, 24-hourly and two-daily cycles as well as the just over 28-day lunar cycle and the cycle of the seasons. In addition to all this, when an equinox comes along it will be able to take advantage of the even higher energies that can facilitate even deeper cleansing at a cellular level.

If we can move with all of these energies and rhythms, we are never going to be stagnant. We are going to be able to detoxify and re-nurture, which are the two fundamental things we need to be able to do in order to maintain health.

Stagnation is an expression of disease. If we want health, we must not allow stagnation to occur in our being on any level. When we get fixed thinking or ideas in our mind, it is a sign of stagnation. When we close our mind, it is a sign of stagnation. A closed mind cuts itself off from all of the influences of the universe. Healing is about creating freedom of movement. Think about how much movement the energies of the universe are trying to bring to bear on our body with these natural rhythms.

The Consequences of Dehydration

We discussed in Chapter 2 how dehydration was the fundamental expression and cause of disease, so let us now look at the consequences of not addressing dehydration. What can we expect to happen if we leave the dehydration alert in place?

Looking at our body as a test tube once again, we know that the conditions within the test tube will have a marked effect on the outcome of any experiment we might conduct in that test tube. For instance, suppose you decided to take some B vitamins. How those B vitamins responded would depend upon the conditions in the test tube. When considering these conditions, the first question we have to ask is, 'Is the test tube hydrated?' We know that if it is not hydrated, then everything will be contracted and therefore not able to move freely.

The next condition we must consider is the pH. We know that when dehydration is present it is going to very much affect the pH. We have already talked about the movement of the four main minerals, sodium and calcium and potassium and magnesium. Where they situate themselves will create the pH in our bodies. When sodium is not properly cleared from a cell at night, the cell remains more acidic, hence the body becomes more acidic. When a body becomes acidic, it is much more prone to disease. Ulcers or arthritis, for instance, can occur only in a body that is too acidic.

Changes in hydration and pH will always affect body temperature. I find that when people have deep stories – by this I mean a long history of disease – they are often-very cold. You notice this particularly in people who have received a diagnosis of serious disease, such as AIDS, and have then been prescribed lots of vaccines. These people have a body temperature that is often markedly below normal. In these circumstances it is quite common for them to have a lot of viral activity going on in their cells. This kind of activity cannot occur in a cell that is hydrated, slightly alkaline and at the correct temperature, as viral activity is created within the cell to correct toxicity.

We know that when the hydration, pH and temperature are not correct, the charge around the cell membrane will also not be correct. As we have seen, there needs to be a marked difference in the charge inside and outside the cell membrane for us to be able to function to our full potential. A strong cell membrane potential gives us energy and vitality. What we find in people with cancer, for instance, is that the charge inside and outside the cell membrane is very similar. This creates a weak potential that means little movement is possible into and out of the cell. This in turn creates a situation of stagnation, and indeed this fits in very neatly with the view of Chinese medicine, which describes cancer as the manifestation of stagnant blood and energy.

I have also had patients with huge electrical sensitivities and allergies, which again is a sure sign that the cell membrane potential has changed. I have even known of patients who have regularly needed to touch something metal, such as a radiator, to earth themselves and discharge electrons that are no longer being held in place around their cell membranes.

We know that the cell membrane potential needs to

be correct for us to be able to hold electron clouds and that it is only when we can hold these clouds around our cells that they can accept and hold photons of light. The changing levels of photon activity that occur during the day and with the changing seasons do not unduly affect people who can hold, produce and utilize light, whereas those whose ability to do so has been compromised may be prone to conditions like SAD.

One of the areas I see most affected by a change in cell membrane potential is fertility. Light is so important for the creation of new life. Fertility is becoming an increasing problem in both animals and humans in our modern world and I know this is intrinsically linked to our ability to hold and use light.

Something we have not discussed so far is the importance of oxygen in our bodies. We all know that we cannot survive without air and the oxygen within it, but what we don't often consider is what happens to the oxygen once it enters our bodies. It has been found that it is the photons and electrons around the cell membrane that attract oxygen and allow the cell to breathe.

Asthma is perhaps the most obvious condition where we see that the oxygen is not able to reach the correct place in the body. Indeed, a high level of body acidity can reduce the body's ability to use oxygen by up to 80 per cent.

Electrons have a great affinity for oxygen, and the electron-rich fats within our bodies are the most oxygen active. So we can see just how vital it is for us to have the correct pH within our cells. Then the electrons, photons and oxygen within us can be utilized to their maximum potential and we can maximize our human potential.

CHAPTER 5

THE PRINCIPLES GUIDING HEALING

It is vital that we learn to work with the body, because it so wants to work with us. To be able to work with the body means understanding the processes it is going through and supporting those processes, particularly when it comes to healing.

Hering's Law

Constantine Hering (1800–1880) was a homoeopath who created a law that was designed for use with homoeopathy, but in all my years of working with patients I have never come across a law that is more succinct or useful in all aspects of healing. It is an amazing way of looking at the effects of treatment and understanding whether one is moving towards or away from healing.

In the healing process there can be times when the body needs to throw off toxicity, and when this happens it is quite common for patients to feel unwell. At these times they are vulnerable to the re-emergence of fears. Questions such as, 'Is this really working?' and 'Am I actually getting worse?' can often rise up in their minds. This is where Hering's Law can be extremely useful, because it gives you a clear indication of whether your current symptoms are a sign of progression or regression.

Hering's Law states:

'Healing takes place from the top to the bottom; from the inside to the outside; from the greater organs to the lesser organs; and in the reverse order in which the dis-ease appeared.'

This means that symptoms will disappear from the head first and the lower parts of the body last, from within the body to the skin, breath and colon, from the more important organs to the less vital ones and in the reverse order in which they first appeared. The true healing process is the reverse of how the dis-ease process manifested.

You can imagine the dis-ease process to be like walking down a forever narrowing corridor. As you walk down this corridor, you accumulate more and more toxicity. When the true healing process begins to take place it is like turning around, going back and revisiting those same levels of toxicity. Fortunately the journey back to health is usually much quicker than the journey towards dis-ease. This is because as you accumulate toxicity, the burden on your body increases and this inevitably slows you down. Conversely, as you release toxicity, you become lighter and freer. When this happens, your journey gathers more and more momentum. Healing is always a journey back to feeling good again. Once you feel good, you can choose new journeys and adventures that will take you into true expansion.

What I often find when a patient is getting better is that as they walk back down that corridor they express the same illnesses that they experienced when manifest-ing their dis-ease process. They are actually experiencing the same imbalance and toxic load that was present at the time the disease first manifested. The information given in the next section, particularly the techniques, will be invalu-able in addressing this imbalance and avoiding discomfort on the journey to health.

We live in a world where the medical profession chops little bits of us off to study, pokes cameras here and there and looks at our blood under microscopes. These are all fragments of the story of who we really are. To heal, we must look at the big picture; we must practise true holism. Samuel Hahnemann, MD (1755–1843), one of the founding fathers of homoeopathy, said that a person's dis-ease was the sum total of what they brought to show you and tell you.

By working with Hering's Law, we can be assured that we will not break any of the natural laws and thus always make progress. So, if disease starts to disappear from the top, what it will touch are the symptoms we express that start with the pronoun 'I'. Patients will say things such as 'I don't feel creative or motivated,' 'I am depressed' and 'I am always tired.' When we use the word 'I', we are expressing thoughts from our higher being, which is the first place to improve when healing is taking place. As healing unfolds, these symptoms will begin to clear, so that the patient might say things such as 'I feel much more hopeful about the future,' 'I can see that it is possible for me to heal' or 'I feel brighter.'

When a patient begins a sentence with the word 'my', they are talking from a much lower place. 'My stomach feels bloated', 'My knee hurts' and 'My back aches' are all signs of a much less serious situation that is more body orientated than head orientated. However, in the dis-ease process, symptoms that are expressed with the prefix 'my' are a sign that the higher aspects of our being are being challenged. If we do not address those symptoms, the disease will inevitably move from the body to the head, from the 'my' to the 'I'.

So often we see someone who in the beginnings of showing arthritis will say that the stiffness is in the end of one of their fingers and then, as the dis-ease progresses, the arthritis moves inwards. It might move to the wrists, then the shoulders, then manifest in the feet and move gradually up the legs and into the hips. Later on it is not uncommon for the dis-ease to move into the body, ultimately affecting the heart and mind.

It is also quite common for a child who has eczema to undergo treatment where the eczema disappears but is replaced by asthma. Here we clearly see that the dis-ease has moved deeper into the body, from a less important organ, the skin, to a more vital organ, the lungs. An illness affecting the lungs is potentially much more life-threatening than one affecting the skin.

This situation can only happen if the treatment has been suppressive. Unfortunately, I see this kind of situation arising from both Western and so-called 'alternative' treatments. Think about how society would change if we taught all of our children Hering's Law. For many children, a visit to see the doctor is like a visit to see a magician. He dishes out his magic potions and 'Hey, presto!' the symptoms are gone. No connection is made when new and more serious symptoms arise. When these too are treated in a suppressive way, the process continues. So it is easy to see how it is that chronic disease is becoming more and more common.

When I was a child, cancer was a rarity. Today it seems that everyone knows of several friends or family members who have died of it. Current treatment of cancer is totally counter to Hering's Law and will never restore true health to an individual. Our Western pharmaceutically driven medicine never really makes us better and ultimately always makes us worse. Health is so much more than a lack of symptoms, it is complete freedom from toxicity, and Hering's Law is a beautiful way of showing us different levels of toxicity.

When you understand Hering's Law you understand the futility of many of the efforts made to improve public health both in the West and abroad. It might seem like a great idea to try to eradicate polio from Africa via mass vaccination, for example, but no one seems to be looking to see whether in fact the vaccination has caused a weakening of the body. Certainly there appears to be no decrease in overall mortality in these mass-vaccinated areas. Quite the contrary in fact, because no sooner is one disease 'eradicated' than a more serious one arises. Just look at the rampant spread of the dis-ease labelled 'AIDS' since its first manifestation.

The Hierarchy of Organs

There is a hierarchy of organs, with the brain and heart being the most important. Dis-ease progresses more deeply into the body by way of this hierarchy, but one can also use this hierarchy to understand the release of dis-ease.

The lowliest organ is the skin. It is also the largest organ in the body. This makes it very useful because if we can get an elimination of toxicity through the skin, it can very often bring great relief to an overburdened body. This release might be by way of sweating, such as happens when a person manifests a fever. When the body produces a fever, the skin becomes the dominant route of elimination. To suppress that fever is to drive the illness deeper into the body.

The next organ in the hierarchy is the colon. Remember that it is the colon that holds the message of whether we are dehydrated or not. An imbalance in the colon feels more uncomfortable to our being than one in the skin.

Next we come to the liver. The liver is the most resilient of our organs. Two-thirds of it can be destroyed and it will still regenerate. It is hugely robust and indeed it needs to be in order for us to survive in the toxic environment we live in these days.

Moving deeper still, we come to the kidneys and the lungs. Notice that we have two of each of these. This is because they are much more delicate and susceptible to damage than the lower organs in the hierarchy. So you can see that if you are supporting the liver, you are also protecting the kidneys and lungs. Interestingly, in the West the skin is considered to be like a third kidney and in the East it is considered to be like a third lung.

Finally within our core are the heart, brain and mind. Lose any one of these and you cannot survive for long. Quite obviously these vital parts of us need all the protection they can get and this protection is provided by the other, progressively more lowly organs. This is why nature absorbs toxicity in this way and releases it in reverse order.

Hering's Law in Operation

So how, for instance, does a child born with a heart imbalance fit into Hering's Law and the hierarchy of organs? In order to understand why this has happened, we need only apply Hering's Law over the previous generations. When we do this we can clearly see how toxicity has accumulated and been passed on from one generation to the next. It is as if the child has been born a long way down that corridor of dis-ease because of the toxicity acquired by its ancestors. This is why in cellular awakening we always look at the predispositions we have brought forward from previous generations.

A person's journey down the corridor of dis-ease is always unique, but Hering's Law will always apply. A typical journey might start with the manifestation of a minor skin disorder. If this is suppressed, it is common for the bowel to show signs of imbalance. This might be constipation or alternating constipation and diarrhoea. There are so many people in the Western world suffering from some form of bowel dysfunction or IBS (irritable bowel syndrome) at the moment. When this is suppressed, we might see problems beginning to arise in the lungs and so on.

When I talk about suppression, I am not talking only about the use of Western drugs to treat symptoms, but also about the rampant use of vaccinations. All vaccines are suppressive by nature. That is what they were designed to do.

I have found that if you vaccinate a healthy child, it will often develop a colon imbalance such as constipation or colic. If you vaccinate a child with a colon imbalance, it will often develop a skin imbalance, like eczema. If you vaccinate a child with a skin imbalance, it will often develop a lung problem. A lung imbalance does not necessarily mean developing full-blown asthma. It might be that the child appears less happy and energetic. Such a child is experiencing a diminution of energy and life force which restricts it from fully expressing its nature and potential. Finally, if the lung imbalance is suppressed, the illness enters the mind. It is becoming very common for a child with lung and colon problems to develop autism after taking the MMR vaccination. The explosion of autism, ADHD and learning problems in our children is a clear indication of just how much toxicity we are passing on to them. This is why I will spend at least two years doing pre-conceptual work with both parents when I treat fertility problems.

It is not only childhood vaccines that create these patterns of dis-ease. As mentioned in Chapter 1, in my practice I have found that in 90 per cent of cases of anorexia that I have treated, the anorexia arose within six months of having the BCG (tuberculosis) vaccine, which in the past often coincided with the onset of puberty. Anorexia is an illness where the toxicity has reached head level.

'Alternative' treatments can also be suppressive. It is not so much about what you are using to help your healing process but *how* you are using it. Even a simple supplement such as magnesium, when applied wrongly, can have a suppressive effect. Furthermore, practices such as counselling, when they focus on problems from the past rather than solutions in the present, can be equally suppressive.

How to Clear the Body of Toxicity

So how can we clear toxicity from the body in a safe and non-suppressive way? This is where what I call 'the art of cellular awakening' becomes so powerful. This is a way of looking at how our cells release toxicity into the lymph, which, as we have seen, then drains into the blood, is filtered by the liver, transported to the bile and excreted out of the body, and how we can support this natural process of healing and rebalancing.

As we journey back down our own unique corridors of dis-ease, it is vital that we release toxicity fully at every level. If the body cannot excrete its toxicity, it will inevitably have to find somewhere else within the body to place it. This is not what we want if we are to return to full health and potential.

To take an example, let us look at how a sore throat might be suppressed and what this might lead to and then follow on with how it might better be treated in a natural way.

When someone has a sore throat, bacterial activity is taking place in order to resolve a toxic situation. Later on we will look at the work of Antoine Béchamp, who showed very clearly how this process works. Basically he revealed that when there is an accumulation of toxicity within the body, the body creates a situation that will facilitate its release. This is known to us as an acute illness. The body will warm itself up and direct extra warmth and blood flow to a particularly toxic area. This warming process has the effect of enabling the release of toxicity, provided the fever is not suppressed while the head is kept cool.

If, however, the sore throat is treated with antibiotics, the whole process is arrested. This means that the congested lymph, which is very much being expressed in the throat, cannot be released. The antibiotics present a new challenge for the body to deal with. This causes stress, which we know leads to dehydration. Antibiotics create more stagnation and because the body cannot release it, the person's story goes a little deeper.

What I often find when looking at a case history involving recurring sore throats, especially in childhood, is that the interval between the sore throats becomes shorter with each course of antibiotics. As the person's story unfolds, though, usually at some point the sore throats disappear.

This often occurs during a transition time such as at the onset of puberty. The illness then begins to manifest at a deeper level, descending to the lungs and manifesting as a lack of energy, an inability to concentrate or a loss of life direction. Perhaps at this time the teenager is labelled as 'difficult'. Subsequently, as the young person matures into adulthood, the disease may have become so deep that it manifests in the mind as depression. The Chinese call the lungs the 'seat of depression', which fits perfectly with our understanding of Hering's Law. By this time it is common to find that the natural cycles of sleep and digestion have become interrupted, further exacerbating the situation. Ultimately, if the depression is further suppressed with medication, the person may well manifest an illness such as ME (sometimes called 'chronic fatigue syndrome'). With ME the person is so stagnant and their lymph so thickened with toxicity that there is no energy available any longer for the body to produce fevers to clear it. This obviously affects the whole vitality and potential of the individual.

If suppression does not take place, the outcome of a sore throat can be very different. In an ideal scenario, as soon as the throat felt uncomfortable, you would address it. You would look at diet, making especially sure to remove all mucous-forming foods, because the lymph would need to become thinner. The diet would also need to become lighter, with a lot more water being added. Next you would support the body's healing process with techniques. A cold damp wrap, for example, placed around the throat, will draw extra energy to that area because the body will naturally want to dry and warm up the cold damp wrap.

If extra energy comes to the throat, this can be utilized to help to resolve the situation. The body uses the heat of a fever to thin the lymph, so suppressing a fever does not make sense. All you need to do is make sure that the head remains cool in order to protect the brain. You might encourage the flow of lymph with other techniques, such as skin brushing (page 161), hot and cold showers (page 164) or even hot tubbing followed by cool wrapping (page 170). When you can get the lymph flowing properly, it will naturally clear the congestion in the throat. You might even aid hydration via the colon with water enemas (page 187), which would further stimulate the flow of lymph.

This kind of management of illness acknowledges that a sore throat is a moment in time involving toxicity and congestion. A return to health means clearing away that toxicity and releasing it from the body. The last thing we need is for the process to be arrested.

There is a general rule regarding acute illnesses. It states that an acute illness will arise three times in the form of a healing crisis (which we will look at later on in this chapter). However, if that illness is suppressed three times, the person's story will go deeper. So you have to ask yourself the next time you hear of a new medicine or vaccination that is supposedly going to make a particular illness disappear, 'Where is that illness really going? Has it truly resolved itself, resulting in the 'I' and human potential improving? Or is it nothing more than another form of suppression that may very well ultimately lead many more people into depression?'

The Difference between Acute and Chronic Illness

Let us take a deeper look at the difference between acute and chronic disease, because it seems to me that in our modern society the distinction between the two is not made.

Chronic Disease

A chronic disease is a condition that has been there for a considerable length of time. It is a manifestation of a chronic toxic load within the body. This chronic load takes up space within the body, space that under normal conditions would be hydrated and free flowing.

People usually demonstrate varying levels of chronic load in different parts of their bodies and we see that the various chronic diseases have their own personalities. These chronic toxic loads are dark, deep and very slow moving, and so tend to create a very cold and acidic environment. A person displaying a high chronic load and manifesting a chronic disease will tend to have a low temperature, an overall acidic pH, be very dry and have cells that are very dark, i.e. lacking in photons.

Examples of chronic diseases include conditions such as asthma, arthritis and the varying syndromes (e.g. ME, multiple sclerosis, Parkinson's and motor neurone disease). None of these diseases can manifest without a chronic toxic load within the body. Perhaps cancer is the deepest disease of them all, but we should also remember that anyone displaying mental illness will also have a very deep picture.

When there is such a large build-up of toxicity within the body it inevitably affects the central nervous system, the endocrine system and of course the electrical charge held within the individual. This lowered charge means that chronic disease pictures usually tend to have within them the manifestation of low energy. I do not just mean low energy for life, but low energy at a cellular level, which inhibits the ability to be able to bring about change.

So how does this chronic load start to build up in the body? The body must always be able to detoxify in order to re-nurture. It needs to be able to throw off what is does not need on a daily basis, but when this process is suppressed and the energy of the body becomes lower, it lays the foundation for the creation of these chronic pictures. Basically the body becomes too cold and dehydrated to produce the energy to create an acute episode.

Toxicity is not only produced as part of our day-to-day living; it can also be inherited. When you look into the health of the parents and grandparents of someone with chronic disease, you can often see an unfolding story of toxic build-up. For instance, the grandparents may have suffered from little more than colds and 'flu when they were growing up. These are acute diseases that enable the body to release toxicity. As they reached their teens they might have had some constipation and a skin problem such as eczema. These kinds of symptoms might be a little inconvenient, but they are not really suppressing the person's potential to any great degree. Remember that the skin is the largest organ of elimination and the lowest in the hierarchy of organs. However, if the eczema is suppressed by the use of allopathic skin creams and drugs, a deeper picture starts to emerge. Toxicity begins to build up and this is then passed on to the next generation. So you might find that one or both of the parents suffered from more chronic diseases during their own childhood, for example recurrent bouts of bronchitis. If these were treated in a suppressive way with repeat doses of antibiotics, then deeper levels of toxicity would build up. We can see here the deepening movement of dis-ease from the skin and colon into the lungs.

A child born to parents who have some form of chronic disease already manifesting prior to conception will come into the world with an inherited chronic load within them from birth. They may well be born, for instance, with asthma, and we know that if this is suppressed by the use of drugs and inhalers the dis-ease will move from the lungs to the mind. This might manifest at some point as depression, behavioural problems or mental illness. Just think how vulnerable a child born to parents with chronic disease is to vaccinations.

When we look at family trees in this way it gives us a beautiful insight into predispositions. Some people are pro vaccination and others against, and there is really no middle ground. However, everybody knows that for some children vaccinations appear to cause little problem, while for others the side effects can be devastating. When you look at the predispositions carried forward in the family line, you can begin to discern which children are the most vulnerable to potential side effects from vaccinations and drugs. This allows parents to make informed choices based upon knowledge rather than fear.

All children these days are born with a level of inherited toxicity, but depending upon how they are raised the chronic load can increase or decrease. The factors we discussed when looking at dehydration, such as diet and lifestyle, start to become very important here. Anyone who has unresolved toxicity will actually be contracted at a cellular level because you cannot have toxicity without dehydration, and dehydration always causes some level of cellular contraction. If a child born with a toxic load is fed a poor diet, has suppressive treatments every time they try to release toxicity and has lots of vaccinations, this is a recipe for serious health problems in adult life.

A chronic illness is the strongest manifestation of dehydration. We know that when we are dehydrated, it is going to cause stress, and that stress will inevitably cause further dehydration. It is within these chronic pictures that we start to see this Catch-22 situation of spiralling levels of dehydration and stress. It is no wonder that these diseases are said to be incurable, but it is a lack of understanding of the way the body truly works that leads to such closed thinking.

So what can we do to bring about positive change in these situations? First we need to understand that when we treat chronic disease, we need to start very gently so that we do not cause further stress and thus drive the disease even deeper within the individual. There will be very little spare energy available in the person and we know that for healing to take place we have to release extra energy, because it is only the body that can heal itself. We also want to be able to create freedom of movement.

The very first thing we need to address is switching off the dehydration alert, because this will immediately stop the disease going any deeper into the body. Then we need to look at the conditions within the test tube. We know that there will be a great deal of unwanted material within that test tube because of the chronic toxic load, so we need next to look at addressing the pH. If we start to rebalance the pH by introducing more alkaline foods, we need to consider what will happen to the acidity that inevitably will be released. Here once again techniques become important to make sure we keep the body's routes of elimination fully open and flowing.

Having begun to address hydration and pH, we then need to look at what is happening to the temperature. A healthy body has the ability to warm itself up and produce an acute episode in order to release toxicity, but people with chronic disease have lost this ability. The obvious answer is to warm them up. Again we have to start gently with something like hot and cold showering, but later on we might be able, for instance, to warm a person up to a temperature of 102°F while keeping the head very cool, in order to allow the lymph to thin and some movement to take place. Often this can create movement in organs and areas where there has been persistent stagnation for many years. Once again this will give rise to a great release of toxicity, so the routes of elimination must be supported.

We also need to address the utilization of light. There are techniques using specific oils than can facilitate this. When we bring more light into the body, we are bringing more information from the macrocosm into the cells, some of which may have been cut off from universal wisdom for many years. The cancer cell, for instance, is completely cut off from universal wisdom, having no electron and photon activity.

Addressing the test tube in this manner creates an unfolding process of releasing toxicity and creating more room. What I find as this process unfolds is that the person gets to a point where they can start to heat up themselves. There is nothing more positive in a person with chronic illness than gaining the ability to create an acute illness. The fever of an acute illness burns away some of the chronic load and so begins to unlock new potential.

Acute Illness

So let us now look more closely at acute illness and its purpose. An acute illness will classically last three days and is normally accompanied by increased heat in the form of a generalized fever or the heating up of a specific area that the body is targeting. This is a sign of an increase in energy that is being focused on a particular part of the body. If you heat anything up, the molecules and even the subatomic particles within it will move more quickly and in the body a fever serves the purpose of speeding the body processes up in order to resolve an imbalance.

An acute illness is in fact a gift that enables a person to become freer at every level and should in no way be suppressed. When it is supported, it creates what is called a 'healing crisis', after which the person will have a lighter toxic load. When it is suppressed, it creates a 'disease crisis', after which the person's toxicity will have travelled even deeper into the body.

Rudolf Steiner said that acute childhood illnesses come about in order for a child to burn off toxicity inherited from the parents. When you vaccinate a child against these acute diseases, you rob that child of the opportunity to become free of inherited toxicity and this has a huge effect on their potential. These flamboyant episodes, whether in childhood or adulthood, only need supporting and managing with what I call 'old-fashioned nursing'.

Acute illnesses involve bacterial activity outside the cell. Now that Western medicine has supposedly eradicated acute illnesses through mass vaccination, what we are now finding is that many chronic illnesses involve viruses acting inside the cell. Viral activity within the cell is far more dangerous and potentially life-threatening than bacterial activity outside the cell.

With the loss of acute illnesses we have seen a loss of human potential and a dramatic increase in chronic 'incurable' diseases. If we want to return to health, we have to look at disease in a way that is different from the accepted medical models, because these models do not work. There has been no overall improvement in the mortality rates for most forms of cancer in the past 100 years, yet still people put their faith in drugs, surgery and radiation. Terminal patients are often offered 'new drugs' in the hope of prolonging life but are in fact being treated as little more than guinea pigs. All disease is curable, but the cure can only be found within the body. When we hand responsibility for our healing to others, we walk further down that narrowing corridor of disease. Perhaps it is time for us to take back our power and to accept our personal responsibility for the care and healing of our own unique vehicles.

Those people who chronically believe that acute illness is 'bad' will find themselves living with chronic disease. Those who dare to think differently, who dare to dream of a return to health and full potential, will find themselves walking back along an ever-widening corridor that leads to happiness, health and freedom.

CHAPTER 6

LASTING GUIDELINES

A Chinese master can sense a disease two years before it manifests in the physical body from the subtle smells emitted by a patient. They can tell which internal organs are feeling most stressed, by the subtle colours around the eyes and the edge of the mouth. Indeed, to a fully trained eye, there are no secrets that we can hold, for our bodies show all imbalances very clearly.

There is a part of the philosophy of Chinese medicine called the 'five element theory' which I find to be the most amazing way of drawing together the sense of connectedness that I talk about. Everything fits into this philosophy because it embraces a total awareness of the expanse of the universe. All of the acupuncture points in Chinese medicine not only have a connection to the body but also

a connection to the universe. From the Chinese perspective we each have the greater universe expressed within
our physical bodies and this understanding brings with it a
great sense of connectedness. The acupuncture meridians
are also pathways through which light travels around our
bodies and we have already seen just how important light
is in our ability to access universal wisdom.

The Consistency of the Five Elements

The five elements of Chinese medicine are Wood, Fire,
Earth, Metal and Water, and each element has many different corresponding and connected aspects, a few of which
we will explore. Each element corresponds to a time of
the year, certain organs and emotions, tastes, smells, sounds
and a whole variety of other aspects.

The five elements can help us to connect at deeper
levels and make sense of what at first might seem unrelat-
ed happenings and feelings. So let us look at each element
individually to see what connections it holds for us.

Wood

The element of Wood corresponds to the time of spring
and the colour green. It has an emotion, which is anger, and
it has organs where this is stored. Everything connected
to the element of Wood is held within the liver and the
gall bladder. The liver has a major function in the body
as 'the planner', so if anything is not going to plan, for
instance wanting to become pregnant, then it is the liver
that needs to be addressed. The liver is the planner for

all of the functions of the body and the gall bladder is 'the decision maker'.

The element of Wood expressed within us can be likened to a tree. We need to have enough flexibility so that we don't break in the winds of change and enough structure so that we are not blown over, so the power of adaptability is strongly linked to this element. If a person has a problem with their structure and flexibility, such as in arthritis, this is regarded as an imbalance in the Wood element. It is also quite common for people with a Wood imbalance to favour the colour green. Each element also has a corresponding orifice and sense organ, which for Wood is the eyes.

In Chapter 4, I mentioned that each organ had a two-hour period when its energy was very focused. The time of the gall bladder is between the hours of 11 p.m. and 1 a.m. The time of the liver follows on from that of the gall bladder and is therefore from 1 to 3 a.m. It is quite common in modern society for people to experience gall bladder problems after eating a fatty meal in the evening. They may go to bed that night and wake up before midnight because they begin to experience gall bladder pain. This often carries on through the times of the gall bladder and liver, so may not subside until after 3 a.m. It is also very common for someone who has a difficult decision to make to find themselves wide awake and unable to sleep until after 1 a.m. because all decision making is connected to the gall bladder. When I meet people who have had their gall bladders removed, it is very interesting to ask them what their decision-making skills are like. Fortunately, even if a person has lost their gall bladder it is still within them energetically and their meridians still function, so healing can still take place.

All these different factors mean that if a person has a problem with their eyes, with their body structure, with their liver and/or gall bladder, if they wake up each night between the hours of 11 p.m. and 3 a.m., if they are prone to anger or if they find the time of spring very challenging, they could have an imbalance of the Wood element.

With this imbalance, as with an imbalance of any of the elements, you would correct the manifestation of dis-ease with cellular awakening and the rebalancing of the element would be addressed by an acupuncturist.

Fire

Wood is what traditionally feeds a fire, so the next element in the five element cycle is Fire. The time of the Fire element is early summer, when the power and strength of the sun are ascending. The emotion of Fire is joy or lack of joy, meaning that someone who is overly happy or overly sad would be regarded as having an imbalance in this element. The colours connected to fire are red and grey, the latter being a lack of the colour red. The orifice of Fire is the ears and the sense organ is the tongue.

There are four organs connected to the Fire element: the heart, the small intestine, the circulation sex and the triple heater. The last two of these organs do not have equivalent organs in Western physiology. The heart is considered to be the 'supreme governor' and the small intestine the 'great separator' of the pure from the impure on all levels of our being.

There are two times of the day linked to Fire. The time of high energy for the heart is between 11 a.m. and 1 p.m. This is followed by the small intestine from 1 to 3 p.m. The time of the circulation sex is from 7 to 9 p.m. and that of the triple heater is from 9 to 11 p.m.

People who want to go out and party every night rather than naturally preparing to follow the day/night cycle and sleep are said to have a Fire imbalance in their triple heater. The triple heater maintains a balance of temperature throughout the body. If you place your hand first on your lower torso (below your navel), then on your middle torso (between your navel and sternum) and then your upper torso (above your sternum), the temperature should feel the same. A person with a triple heater imbalance often finds that there is a noticeable difference between the temperature of these three regions.

Earth

When a fire burns it creates ash, which becomes earth, so the next element in the cycle is Earth. Earth corresponds to the time of late summer when all the fruits are ripening. The colour is yellow and the emotion is sympathy or empathy. The orifice is the mouth. It has a further important connection, and that is to the energy of mothering. This means both our connection to Mother Earth and our connection to our physical mother. It also connects to our own ability to mother, whether we are male or female, which means our ability to nurture ourselves and others.

The organs of the Earth element are the stomach and spleen.

The time of day of the stomach is from 7 to 9 a.m. and this is followed by that of the spleen from 9 to 11 a.m.

In the East it is common for breakfast to be the largest meal of the day because it is eaten at the time of high energy for the stomach. Eating a large meal at night, especially after dark, puts stress on the stomach at a time when it is not at its most vital. If the stomach cannot process an overabundance of food, that food will tend to remain in it and can cause problems such as heartburn and acid reflux.

Metal

The Earth is the source of minerals and ores, so the next element is Metal, which corresponds to the time of autumn. The colour is white and the emotion is grief. This is not only grief for what has been but also for what might have been. The organs of Metal are the colon, skin, lungs and mind, and within this element is the energy of 'seeking perfection'. A further connection is with the energy of fathering, which encompasses how you view your spirituality (the 'heavenly father') and your own earthly father. It is also connected to your ability to father, whether you are male or female.

The skin and mind work continuously, so do not have their own appointed times of high energy, but the peak time of the lungs is from 3 to 5 a.m. and the time of the colon is from 5 to 7 a.m. This means that if a person frequently wakes up at 3 a.m. and cannot get back to sleep until 5 a.m., there will be some connection to the energy of the lungs. The orifice and sense organ of the Metal element is the nose.

Water

In ancient China mirrors were made from metal and if a metal mirror was left out overnight it would attract dew to its surface, so the final element in our cycle is Water. Winter is the time of the Water element and the colours connected to it are blue and black. The emotion is fear and the organs are the kidneys and bladder. The orifices are the anus and urethra and the sense organ is the ears. The time of the bladder is from 3 to 5 p.m. and the time of the kidneys is from 5 to 7 p.m.

Wood depends upon water for its ability to grow, so we see that the element of Water gives birth to the element of Wood and thus the cycle of the five elements and the cycle of the year as depicted by the five elements is complete.

There are also many further connections involved in the five elements, such as different sounds of voice, different qualities of dreams and different food preferences.

An Example of How the Elements Can Become Imbalanced

Let us look now at a theoretical case history to see the five elements in action.

Imagine a baby girl that is born by Caesarean section. The liver of the mother would have planned for a normal birth and the decision of when to initiate the birth would have been the responsibility of her gall bladder. A Caesarean section overrides these natural processes and that could mean that the child is born with an imbalance in the Wood element (the element of the liver and gall bladder), passed on from the mother.

If that baby is vaccinated in the manner current in our society, she might receive 32 different vaccines in the first two years of her life. Subjecting a new life to the resonance of 32 different diseases will inevitably create stress and, as we have already seen, stress causes dehydration, so the Water element will now also become imbalanced.

Now suppose that as this child grows up, she is bullied at school. This will add further stress and dehydration, but will also bring about a lack of joy, which in turn brings the Fire element into play.

Then perhaps in early adulthood the dehydration reaches a level where it affects the functioning of the colon, so constipation becomes a part of this young woman's picture and this brings the Metal element into play. Then suppose she experiences the death of her father. The Metal element is not only connected to the colon but also to grief and the energy of the father. This bereavement has the potential to cause a deepening of the Metal imbalance.

As our imaginary person reaches her early thirties, perhaps she has an attack of colitis in the autumn. When you understand the five elements this is no surprise, because the Metal element corresponds to both the colon and the time of autumn. In my practice I frequently find that when taking a case history of someone with colon problems, their first attack occurred shortly after the autumn equinox. In this fictitious case history, the colitis is suppressed with drugs, sending the dis-ease deeper into the Metal element, and this is manifested as bronchitis in the woman's forties. This is further suppressed with medication, taking both the Metal and Water pictures even deeper.

As this woman reaches her menopause, a time of major transition, the stress of menopausal symptoms means that the level of dehydration becomes so deep that hypertension arises, which is linked to the kidneys and Water element. If medication is given, this adds further to the dehydration.

The next symptom that arises is abdominal pain when going to bed after eating late in the evening, and gall stones are diagnosed. Here the Wood element has arisen once again.

As we move into this woman's sixties, we find arthritis showing up, with stiffness and pain. This will be a combination of the Wood and Water elements showing further imbalance. As this woman reaches her late sixties, the level of dehydration and imbalance is so deep that her body is no longer able to defend the most vital of organs and she has a heart attack. Once again the Fire element shows itself.

If we were to look closely at the food preferences at different times in this woman's life, they would most likely be linked to the elemental imbalance showing at that time. When we look later on at actual case histories (see

Appendix I), we will see more clearly how the five elements philosophy helps to give a deeper understanding of an unfolding story of dis-ease within a person.

Honouring Ancestral Predispositions

There is a pattern of imbalance in the Metal element that I have come across again and again in my practice and I call this pattern the 'tubercular taint'. During my many years of practising and teaching I have noticed that there is a great disparity between what is written down in books and what I actually find in my clinical practice. For instance, many authors say that the omega 3 essential fatty acid has amazing curative properties for many diseases, such as type 2 diabetes and bipolar disease, but I have met people who have taken omega 3 and not experienced any positive benefits. I realized many years ago that this must be due to the conditions in the test tube and a pattern began to reveal itself to me. When certain things have occurred generation after generation in a person's family line, I find that the conditions within that person's test tube are no longer conducive to effectively utilizing oils such as omega 3. I do agree that omega 3 has life-changing potential, but only when the conditions within the test tube are correct.

So what exactly is the tubercular taint? It is an energetic blueprint that is passed down through the generations. For instance, if there is nutritional deprivation in a group of people, resulting in failing health, there will be changes within their bodies. When these people reproduce, those changes will be passed on to the next generation via this energetic blueprint. If these deficiencies are not addressed by that generation, the blueprint carries forward along the family line. This explains why so many people I meet have such deep pictures. These deeper pictures are manifested as our illness predispositions, so although we may be living longer there are so many more chronic conditions, for example ME, autism, MS and myriad bowel diseases which cause much suffering.

If we look at the west coast of Ireland during the potato famine, for example, we see that many of the starving population contracted tuberculosis (TB). Today we find that the people living in this area have one of the highest incidences of coeliac disease and that if not treated correctly it can lead to schizophrenia. However, I have realized that it is not possible for a person who is born healthy to manifest schizophrenia in just one generation. For schizophrenia to come about there has to have been a preceding pattern, and part of this pattern often involves the contraction of TB by the previous generations.

So what exactly is the imbalance that arises from TB? TB is a manifestation of the inability to keep calcium in the correct place within the body. In Chapter 2 we saw just how important calcium was in the day/night cycle and that if the night-time cleanse was not completed, both sodium and calcium remained within the cell when they should be outside the cell. In this situation we would say that the sodium and calcium were misplaced. The misplacement of calcium within the body is the result of dehydration, but it is also linked to imbalances within the blood sugar, because the moment calcium is misplaced, energy levels will start to drop. The misplacement of calcium can become progressively worse generation after generation, so what started in one generation as an inability to cleanse the cell leads to a more imbalanced situation in the next generations. As the generations unfold, there is a change in hydration, pH, temperature and the ability to utilize light, and there is a progressive inability to keep calcium in the correct place within the body.

When I look at a case history, one of the first things I look for are signs of this tubercular taint. I find that in a majority of the deep pictures, such as with ME, infertility, Crohn's disease and schizophrenia, there is this tubercular picture, this inability to correctly place calcium, within the family history. Indeed, it is quite common for such people to have knowledge of TB occurring within their ancestry.

I have found that peoples from certain parts of the globe are more predisposed to have this taint, especially those of Celtic or Jewish origin. However, any indigenous people who have migrated, either voluntarily or forcibly, to a place where they can no longer obtain the correct balance of essential fatty acids can be prone to this. I see it especially in people from places such as Glasgow and Liverpool in the UK whose ancestors formerly lived on the coastal regions of Ireland and ate a fish-rich diet. Once these people moved inland and stopped eating fish, they became deficient in essential fatty acids.

When the tubercular taint is present within a person's blueprint, certain processes within the body, such as the correct utilization of oils, are impaired. What I have also found in my clinical practice is that the stronger the tubercular taint is within a family, the more changes there are in the structure of the jaw. During the gestational period, the two sides of the jaw should come together quite early on and push down to form a normal wide bite between the teeth. When the tubercular taint is present, however, the two sides of the jaw come together late, resulting in a tighter jaw shape which leads to overcrowding of the teeth. In the most extreme cases this actually leads to the formation of a cleft palate and hairlip.

As well as these changes in the jaw, you also see changes in the shape of the occipital area, which is something I have found repeatedly in people suffering from ME. A high roof to the mouth and an improper bite at the back of the teeth in a baby often also results in problems weaning, due to interruption of the swallowing reflex.

Some beautiful work was carried out in the early part of the last century by Dr Weston Price, who studied indigenous people around the world to see the effect of the adoption of a diet of refined sugar, flour and other processed foods on their health. The people he studied traditionally ate meat or fish regularly in their diet. When people eat animal produce, the animal will have already broken down the parent omega 3 and omega 6 into DHA and Arachidonic acid, so people who traditionally eat an animal-based diet will not have need of the ability to break parent omega 3 and 6 down.

When Weston Price was called to the bedside of a person who was dying, he would drip melted butter and cod liver oil into their mouths and they would invariably recover. The butter had to be made from milk that had been taken from the cow in the spring or the autumn, because at these times the cow would feed on fresh lush grass. Fresh grass is rich in parent omega 6, which the cow would convert into Arachidonic acid. So what Weston Price was actually doing was giving these patients broken-down omega 3 (from the cod liver oil) and broken-down omega 6 (from the butter). We saw in Chapter 3 how the body breaks down parent omega 3 and omega 6 by inserting extra double-carbon bonds and it does this with the help of an enzyme called Delta-6-desaturase, or D6D. This enzyme must be present in the body for us to be able to break down both parent omega 3 and omega 6.

What Weston Price found was that when people who traditionally ate animal produce adopted a Western diet of processed foods and oils, they developed health problems and their offspring had malformed jaws. It seems that their bodies had become so used to obtaining omega 3 and omega 6 in broken-down form from their animal produce that D6D wasn't being made. Hence when they stopped eating their traditional diet, they became deficient in essential fatty acids, even though there was often plenty of parent omega 3 and omega 6 in their diets.

What I have found in my own practice is that in order for the body to be able to produce D6D, hydration, pH and temperature must all be correct, but the body must also have a good supply of magnesium, zinc, omega 3, omega 6 and vitamins B3, B6, C and E. These are exactly what it needs to produce prostaglandins, as we saw in Chapter 3. So you can see that we each need the conditions in our test tube to be correct and to have the correct nutrition if we are to be able to utilize oils correctly.

Going back to look at the people who lived on the west coast of Ireland, traditionally they would have eaten fish and butter and therefore would have had an ample supply of essential fatty acids in their broken-down form. However, during times of famine, because they would probably not hold D6D in their bodies and would not be able to consume the right foods at that time to make D6D, it is no wonder that their health began to fail. It is also little surprise that the next generations were born with the inability to utilize oils. Coeliac disease, which is a disease where gluten in the diet cannot be tolerated, can always be traced back to an initial inability to effectively break down oils. What's more, if this problem is not addressed, it will all too often progress to schizophrenia. This should not be a surprise, because we know how vital broken-down omega 3 and 6 are for the brain and central nervous system. This is why we see that for some people, taking omega 3 brings about a dramatic improvement in health whereas for others it appears to have no effect.

Depression and the Ability to Utilize Oils

In Chinese medicine mental illness is connected to the Metal element and indeed the tubercular taint is also very connected to the Metal element. The Metal element governs the skin, colon, lungs and mind. The lungs are also regarded as the seat of depression. We also know that depression is connected to our ability to utilize light. If a person is unable to make D6D, they will be unable to break down oils, and if they cannot break down oils, then they are not going to be able to form electron clouds around the cell membrane. Equally, if a person cannot keep calcium in the correct place, they will not be able to maintain the correct charge around the cell membrane. Remember that the outer side of the cell membrane needs to have a strong positive charge in order to attract the negatively charged electrons and thus be able to accept the photons of light. You can see how important it is to reawaken this pathway in people with depression, especially when you consider that it might have become blocked three or more generations ago.

There is no point in suggesting to people with depression that they take oils if they cannot metabolize those oils effectively. It is the same with people who suffer from SAD (seasonal affective disorder), because these people need not only to be able to utilize light more effectively but also to be able to hold that light around each cell.

If we look at the mind in connection to this understanding of light and oils, we can see that so many of the mental problems in our society today have their root in this inability to store and utilize light. This not only includes mental illness, but also addictions and destructive thought patterns. Remember that the brain needs the four double-carbon bonds of Arachidonic acid and the six double-carbon bonds of DHA in order to function fully.

What I have also found is that if a person cannot utilize oils, then they will also be unable to utilize zinc. In the addictive and obsessive person, there is always an imbalance in the zinc/copper ratio within the body in favour of copper. However, once again one cannot redress this balance until one has first addressed the utilization of oils. This means making sure that the person can make D6D.

Arachidonic acid is not only used in the brain but is also a vital constituent of one of the main groups of prostaglandins, known as prostaglandins 1. One of the most important functions of these particular tissue hormones is keeping calcium in the correct place within the body, so you can see how everything is interconnected to our ability to utilize oils correctly. If calcium is not in the correct place, blood sugar will not be stable and therefore there will not be the energy available for a person to heal.

If you look back at the actual treatment of TB in the past, you will find that the best treatment took place up in the mountains where there was very clear air and pure light.

The Pasteur/Béchamp Mistake

So many of our modern chronic diseases are connected to this tubercular aspect, because if we cannot break down oils effectively it has a knock-on effect on our central nervous systems, our endocrine systems and all the cells of our bodies.

You can begin to see that the modern medical idea that we catch illnesses from bacteria and viruses is fundamentally flawed. The idea that we are susceptible to attack from microbes was put forward by Louis Pasteur. He said that disease was caused by something outside the human body invading it. These invaders were called bacteria, and from this theory came the idea that to cure disease one only had to kill the bacteria. When Fleming discovered penicillin it was hailed as the end of all disease and since then more and more antibiotics have been produced to kill these invaders. The problem is that far from eradicating disease, antibiotics have created new and more complex diseases. Bacterial activity takes place outside the cell and, as we have seen, is part of the body's way of releasing toxicity. If you arrest that process, the illness must go deeper and this is why we now see so much more viral activity occurring inside the cell.

Why is it that you can have a bus filled with people who are all exposed to many different bacteria in the air and on the seats and yet few if any go on to develop an infection? The only logical conclusion is that it is what is going on within the body of each individual that dictates whether illness manifests or not. This is what a man called Antoine Béchamp realized at the same time that Pasteur was promoting his theory. Béchamp sought to share his own view with the world, but unfortunately Pasteur's ideas, which he himself repudiated when on his deathbed, had already taken hold.

Sadly, Western medicine still holds firm to the belief that illness is caused by an outside invasion, even though so many chronic diseases cannot be linked to the activity of microbes. It is even highly questionable whether the syndrome known as AIDS is caused by an outside invasion, especially when you consider that the HIV virus has never actually been isolated. Dr Douglas Lewis of the Pasteur Institute in Seattle, USA, has done a great deal of work with AIDS patients, and he found that AIDS can only manifest in a person with a lower than normal body temperature. Once again we see that it is really the conditions in the test tube that we must consider. In my own work I have found that anyone taking antibiotics will have, as a side effect, a drop in body temperature. An important part of Douglas Lewis's effective treatment of AIDS involved heating his patients up twice a week in order to create a fever.

The accepted theory of AIDS is that it is caused by a virus. Even if this is true, we have to ask ourselves whether the person caught the virus, whether it was already within the cell and became active only under the right circumstances or whether it was actually created by the conditions within the cell. The theories of Pasteur have no answer to these questions. Perhaps a deeper look at the work of Béchamp might provide us with a clearer picture.

Béchamp said that all manifestations of disease occurred because of what was present within a person, not what was outside them. This makes so much sense even in the simplest way when you consider the people on the bus exposed to supposedly infectious pathogens. If a person on the bus did go on to develop an infection, you have to ask what was lacking in them in order for them to succumb to that infection?

Béchamp found that there were micro-organisms within the body, which he called microzymes, that would change form depending upon the environment that they were in. It was the body environment that dictated the form and the purpose of their activity. Put simply, when the environment outside the cell needs cleansing, you have bacterial activity. When this natural process is arrested with allopathic treatments such as antibiotics, the toxicity moves to deeper within the cell. So then, in order to cleanse the environment inside the cell, you have the awakening of viral activity inside the cell. Viral activity occurs in order to bring about change; it is created by the cell in order to enable it to detoxify. However, it is a situation that only arises when the toxic load within the body becomes too great for bacterial activity to be possible.

One of the most exciting things about my work is finding connections. Most people would not link colon problems with mental illness, but when you understand how the five elements work and connect that understanding with the works of Antoine Béchamp and Constantine Hering, the link is obvious and highly significant. And when you can give a patient a clear picture of how their illness came to exist and flourish, they immediately see their path back to wellness.

Through an understanding of the interconnectedness of everything in our amazing universe, we can make the connection back to our inner wisdom. When we work with nature, she guides us clearly on a path to feeling and being well. This means eating and living as naturally as possible and dancing with all of the universal rhythms. When we achieve this, we become true creators of our own reality with a deep inner knowing of who we are and why we are here.

The next section of the book shows how you can apply this information in a gentle way to yourself and come to fit into and feel at peace with the natural dance of life.

PART II

How We Can Help Ourselves to Dance to Nature's Rhythms

CHAPTER 7

EMPOWER YOURSELF FROM YOUR OWN STORY

Everything in the universe is connected; nothing happens in isolation and nothing happens by chance. Once you understand how the body works and how it responds to the natural rhythms of the universe, there is a sense of wonder at its amazing integrity. Symptoms become signs of an unfolding and reversible pattern rather than isolated incidents and random sabotage. We are all unique and wonderful individuals and we all have our own story to tell. Even two people with the same named disease will have taken very different paths to creating it.

For most doctors and practitioners, taking a case history is a means of understanding a person's story, but if a person cannot understand their own story they will not be able find true health. However, when a case history is properly taken and then has the principles discussed in Part I applied to it, many connections begin to fall into place. As this unfolds, a person begins to see how their current health fits into a bigger picture.

When you understand your own story, the mystery of illness evaporates and with it the fear of future ill health. When you understand that your body is always your friend and that it guides you through your feelings, you will have all you need to find perfect health. Remember, the body *never* works against you and *always* does the very best it can for you at any given point in time.

Healing is about creating freedom and movement. The only thing that stops movement is fear, so whatever releases fear promotes healing. Things that make you feel good release fear and things that make you feel bad increase fear, so if you trust your feelings and do only those things that feel good, you will walk a gentle path back to health and connectedness. You are the only person who can heal yourself because you are the only person holding the knowledge of who you really are.

When discovering your own story, a good place to begin is where you are right here and now, so we will begin the case history with questions about the present. We will take a tour through the body from top to bottom, noticing how different parts feel. Then we will look at your life chronologically from birth through to the present. Next we will take the story deeper by looking at the health of your parents and grandparents, as well as any other significant relatives, and finally we will look at your diet. This will connect you with a lot of information, some of which you might have forgotten until now. Once you have taken your own case history, we will apply our principles to it and you will begin to fit your story into the wider picture.

For this exercise you will need a pen, several sheets of paper and an hour during which you will not be disturbed. Some people even find it useful to unplug or turn off their telephone while doing this.

So let us discover your story.

Your Case History

What Is Presenting Itself in your Story Now?

Write down any aspects of your life that are currently troubling you. This might be health problems or areas of your life about which you feel unhappy or stuck.

Write down also how you would like your life to be. How would you like to feel? What kind of job would you like to have? What kind of relationship do you want? If we want to be happy, healthy and free we have to dare to dream and then walk towards that dream. Cellular awakening is all about connecting to the part of yourself that knows how to manifest your dream life.

Touring the Body from Top to Bottom
The Higher Self
- What are your levels of motivation and creativity?

This does not necessarily mean being an artist or involved in some other form of creative pursuit; it is connected to your ability to think creatively and be motivated. When the higher self is engaged, our creativity finds solutions to all our problems and we have the motivation and determination to realize our dreams. These two key aspects are often the first to decrease as a person moves from good health to illness.

The Mental/Emotional Level
- Do you have any mental or emotional problems?

This is asking whether you are predominantly happy or sad. Do you often have fears, worries or anxieties? Do you ever feel angry, guilty or stressed? How easy is it for you to change from feeling bad to feeling good? Do you have trouble letting go of the past?

Energy Levels
- How are your energy levels?

You can assess your energy levels by comparing them to those of other people or to how you have felt in the past. Make a note of any differences in energy levels throughout the day. Does your energy dip at any time? Do your energy levels improve or diminish depending on the season?

Concentration and Memory
- Is your concentration good?
- How are your long-term and short-term memory?

This question is linked to your brain and central nervous system and gives an indication of how much light you are holding.

Sleep
- Do you find sleep refreshing?
- Do you have difficulty getting to sleep?
- Are there any patterns of waking up and falling asleep?
- Do you wake at specific times during the night?
- How often do you wake up to go to the toilet?
- Is your sleep restless?
- Does the moon (especially the full moon) influence your sleep?

Hair and Scalp
- Is your hair dry or greasy?
- Do you have brittle or falling hair?
- Have there been any changes to your hair, e.g. texture?
- Does your scalp flake or itch?

Skin and Nails

- Is your skin dry or greasy?
- Do you have any rashes or eruptions?
- Does your skin itch?
- Is your skin particularly sensitive?
- Are your nails soft, dry or flaky?
- Do your nails grow quickly?
- Do your nails break easily?

Headaches

If you get headaches:

- How often?
- When are they most likely to occur (e.g. on waking, in front of a computer)?
- Where in the head is the pain?
- Are they accompanied by nausea or vomiting (especially with migraines)?
- Do you notice any other symptoms (e.g. no urination before the onset of a migraine)?

Sinuses

- Do you have any sinus problems, perhaps seasonally (e.g. hay fever)?
- Do you have post-nasal drip as a result of sinus problems?
- Do you experience pressure in your sinuses?
- Do you have blockages affecting your ears or leading to headaches?
- Do you snore?

Eyes
- Do you have any vision problems?
- Do you suffer from eye infections?

Ears, Nose and Throat
- Do you have problems with ear infections internally or externally?
- Do you suffer from tinnitus?
- Does anything affect the quality of your hearing?
- Do you produce a lot of ear wax?
- Do you have any nasal problems with physical blockages (polyps, deformities)?
- Do you get many colds or discharges from the nose?
- Do you get many throat infections and if so, what influences this (e.g. you may get sore throats every three weeks or when you are particularly tired or run down)?
- Do your glands swell up if you get a sore throat?

Mouth and Teeth
- Do you get mouth infections (e.g. ulcers, herpes)?
- Do you have gingivitis or gum problems?
- Do you have overcrowded teeth?
- Do you have a particularly high roof to your mouth or problems with your bite?
- Do you have fillings? If so, do you have a mixture of metals in your mouth (e.g. gold and amalgam)?
- Do you have dentures?
- Do you have root canal fillings?

Lungs

- Do you get lung infections?
- Do you have breathing problems?
- Are you a deep or shallow breather?
- Do you exercise freely?
- Do you regularly produce mucous from your lungs?

Digestion, Stomach and Upwards

- Do you get stomach upsets or periods of nausea and/or vomiting?
- Do you belch or have acid reflux? If so, what influences this?
- Do you have a slow or quick digestion?
- Do you get bloating (particularly after eating or at the end of the day)?

Bowels

- How often do you open your bowels?
- Does a bowel evacuation feel complete?
- Is there any pain when opening your bowels?
- Is there any mucous or blood in your stools? If so, what colour?
- What shape is your stool? Does it float or sink? Is it loose or compact?
- Do you get diarrhoea or constipation?

Urination

- What is the pattern and frequency of your urination (both day and night)?

- Do you get discomfort or retention of urine?
- Does your urine feel acidic or burning?
- Do you have cystitis or nephritis?
- Are you incontinent?
- What are the colour and odour of your urine?
- Is there mucous or blood in your urine?

Menstruation (if appropriate)

- Are your periods regular and what is the length of your cycle?
- Are your periods heavy, painful or clotted?
- How many days does your period last?
- Do you get PMS? If so, what are the associated symptoms (e.g. pains, bloating or depression) and how long do they last?

Aches and Pains (in muscles and joints)

- Describe any aches and pains in detail.
- Where are they situated?
- How long have they been there?
- What makes them better or worse?
- Is the pain permanent or intermittent?
- Do you have swelling?
- Do aches and pains impede activities?

Looking at your Life Picture Chronologically
Going Back to Birth

- How old was your mother at the time of your birth?

- What is your position in the family in relation to other siblings? What is the age gap between siblings?
- Did your mother have any miscarriages or terminations, particularly before your conception?
- Did your mother have any difficulty in conceiving?
- What was your mother's health like during her pregnancy?
- What was your birth like? Was it a natural birth or a Caesarean or forceps delivery?
- Was the pregnancy full term? If premature, were you in an incubator for a period?
- What was your birth weight?
- Were you breast or bottle fed?
- If bottle fed, were there any complications due to allergies?

Infancy (up to two years of age)

- Were you vaccinated in infancy?
- How was your health during your infancy? Were there any issues around thriving, feeding problems, skin health or ENT (ear, nose and throat) health?
- Did you sleep well?
- Did you have any surgery?
- What was your diet like during infancy?
- Did you have any developmental problems in infancy (e.g. slow talking, walking, potty training, ability to play)?
- Did you have any problems with teething or weaning?
- Did you have any accidents?

Childhood (three years up to teens)

- Did you have any vaccinations during this time?
- What illnesses did you have (e.g. measles, chickenpox, mumps)?
- How was your general health (e.g. skin, bowels, appetite)?
- Did you sleep well?
- Did you have any surgery?
- What was your diet like?
- Did you have any learning or behavioural problems (e.g. dyslexia, disruptive behaviour or an inability to sit, listen or concentrate)?
- Were you colour-blind?
- Did you have any autistic-like behaviour?
- Did you have any accidents?

Teens

- Did you have any vaccinations (especially the BCG/TB vaccination)?
- When was the onset of puberty (note the closeness to any BCG vaccination)?
- Did you have any illnesses and how were they treated (e.g. glandular fever, acne, asthma)?
- Did you have any surgery?
- Did you have any eating disorders?
- Did you have any behavioural or learning problems (e.g. depressive behaviour, especially around the pressure of exams)?

- Did any addictive behaviour arise (e.g. excessive smoking, drinking, eating or social drugs)?
- Were there any particular problems associated with puberty (e.g. if male, undescended testicles; if female, absence of periods)?
- If female, was any form of contraception used?
- Were there any problems with sleep or with normal functioning generally?
- What kind of diet did you eat?
- Did you have any accidents?

Decade by Decade to the Present Time

- Did you have any vaccinations (e.g. for travel abroad or because of work) and were there any reactions to these?
- Did you have any illnesses? If so, how were they treated and what was the outcome?
- Did you have any surgery?
- If female, did you use any form of contraception?
- Was there any addictive behaviour or were there mental or emotional problems?
- Did you have any sustained bouts of stress?
- If female, did you have any pregnancies? If so, what were they like?
- If female, did you have any pregnancy terminations or miscarriages?
- Did you have any accidents?
- What kind of diet did you eat?

Family Patterns
Parents' Health
- Where were your parents born?
- What illnesses have your parents suffered? How have these been treated?
- If your parents are deceased, what was the cause of death and at what age?
- Note anything else that may be relevant to your story.

Grandparents' Health
- Where were your maternal and paternal grandparents born?
- What illnesses have your grandparents suffered? How have these been treated?
- If your grandparents are deceased, what was the cause of death and at what age?
- Note anything else that may be relevant to your story.

Your Children
- Note any illnesses or other information that may be relevant.

Any Other Relatives (if relevant)
- Where were they born?
- What illnesses have they suffered? How have these been treated?
- If they are deceased, what was the cause of death and at what age?

Diet

- What is a typical day's nutrition for you (food and drink)?
- How much alcohol, tea or coffee do you drink?
- Do you smoke? If so, how much?
- Do you take any social drugs, supplements or prescribed drugs?

Make a note of any other relevant information.

How to Interpret your Case History

To be well and empowered we need to be fully connected to all the unfolding energies in our universe. If we live in a very disconnected world, it becomes very difficult to find the solutions to our problems. Think of someone having, for instance, a sore throat every three months. If they disconnect that from everything else that is going on around their health picture, it will be very difficult to understand why this is happening and to be able to do anything about it. Everything sits within a pattern and nothing happens in isolation, though all too often symptoms are viewed with no connection to what has gone on in the past. When you do not consider *how* and *why* a symptom has manifested and when you do not connect it with everything else that has been unfolding in your life, the past will repeat itself, and with each repetition the disease will go deeper. To seek only to eradicate symptoms is to disconnect further from who we really are.

Remember that the body never works against us but has perfect integrity, so that it always does the very best it can for us at any given point in time and is always seeking to return to balance. The adaptations it makes are designed to keep us alive, even if we perceive them as degeneration. When we understand how and why our body has adapted, we can implement changes in the way we live in order to make that adaptation obsolete. When the body no longer needs to adapt, for instance to dehydration, it will switch off its dehydration alert and every cell will shine more brightly as a result.

An integral purpose of connecting your story is personal empowerment and the reduction of fear. We each need to rise above the situation we find ourselves in so as to be able to see the fastest and easiest route to manifesting a new and improved situation, but we also need the power and motivation to embrace that path.

The only thing that stops us doing anything, including getting better, is fear. When we connect the different elements of our own story, when we begin to understand the *how* and *why*, there will automatically be a reduction of fear. When people are very ill, they tend to become trapped in a cocoon of fear and find it very difficult to find the answers they need in order to get out of that situation. Often all they can see is a stream of negative events. But when we look at past events with the intent of connecting and understanding, the story begins to change.

How we connect is by applying all of the principles we discussed in Part I to our own story and feeling which of them resonate with what we are seeing now. Each time a new connection is made, there will be a deepening of understanding and a reduction of fear. This will create movement on all levels.

Nothing ever happens by chance. We hear of somebody 'suddenly' becoming ill, but this is just not possible. As already mentioned, a good traditional Chinese doctor knows that illness can be perceived energetically two years before it manifests physically. As a person gets closer to the manifestation of an illness, their body shows many signs, such as a change of mood and emotion, a change of body smell and a change of the character of the voice, which each have their significance. Everything that happens is part of a connected story, and by asking the right questions we can begin to understand our own unique part of that story and to see a bigger picture. By the end of the interpretation there should be a noticeable shift in the energy body and the physical body will respond to this shift. There will be a raising of vibration and with it will come new possibilities for change.

INTERPRETATION KEY

The Higher Self	How connected are we to our full potential?
The Mental/Emotional Level	Depression is often linked with brain dehydration and an inability to store light in the electron clouds. The different emotional problems are linked to the specific organs related to the five elements, e.g. anger, the liver; grief, the lungs; see page 90.
Energy Levels	These give a clear picture of the consistency of the blood sugar. Dips at certain times pinpoint specific organs (see the organ times related to the five elements, page 90).
Concentration and Memory	These are linked to the central nervous system with its great need for constant blood sugar and double-carbon bonds of essential fatty acids for light utilization.
Sleep	See the pattern of waking at certain times or problems at certain times linked to organ times, e.g. waking always at 3–5 a.m. equals the lungs showing up.
Hair and Scalp, Skin and Nails	The hair is a strong indicator of kidney function and the hydration levels, also the thyroid function.
Headaches	Where they occur in the head shows up different acupuncture meridians that are linked to specific organs, e.g. corner of eyes (close to nose) = the bladder meridian. The times of the headaches can again be linked to organ times, indicating which organs are struggling.
Sinuses	The sinuses are the outer part of the lungs with the nose, so indicate where work needs to be done. The sinuses are often linked to depression and the lungs are the seat of depression.
Eyes	The eyes are the orifice of the liver, so any symptoms may show a need to treat the liver. They also often show misplaced fluids – dry eyes = excess fluid elsewhere.
Ears	Ear problems often show in children. They can also be an outer manifestation that care needs to be taken with hydration and the kidneys.
Nose	The nose is an outward sign of the lungs and also indicates thickened lymph when there are mucous congestion problems.
Throat	The throat shows very quickly any dehydration, particularly in young people. The dryness is causing stagnant lymph and the lymphatic tonsil tissue responds, also the lymph nodes. The throat can be quite a barometer of health.
Mouth and Teeth	Each tooth is connected to a different meridian, so reflects the conditions of the organ served by that meridian.

Lungs	The lungs are related to the intake of chi and known as the seat of depression. The breathing levels are also involved in controlling the body pH.
Digestion, Stomach and Upwards	These show the connection with nurturing and the mother and Mother Earth (as shown in the five elements system).
Bowels	The great indicator of hydration levels and therefore connected to how well skin, lungs and mind can function.
Urination	The changing pH of the body will be shown up in the urination habits and experience. Hydration can also be noticed with urination patterns. The Water element and the fear levels are very connected, therefore also connected to the central nervous system.
Menstruation	Linked to liver function, as the planner of the body decides the regularity. If overloaded, the liver also influences menstruation. It can make periods unduly heavy or maybe create fibroids (often called a secondary liver).
Aches and Pains in Muscles and Joints	The problem can be located by checking the meridians involved and therefore the organ connection. Arthritic-type aching always involves Wood and Water, liver and kidneys.

When looking at different principles relating to our case history, we need to apply them chronologically so that we can see our story unfolding. So let us now look at these principles one by one to see how they fit into your own story.

1. The Dehydration Alert

The first principle is the dehydration alert. When the body becomes dehydrated, it starts to make cellular changes as a means of defence. So what kind of things are we likely to notice within our story as indicators of dehydration?

The first thing that takes place when dehydration arises is a disconnection from the higher aspects of ourselves. This can manifest as a loss of direction in life, an inability to escape from a repeatedly stressful situation or a loss of creativity and motivation. For some people it can mean having enough energy to go to work during the day but then being so tired and unmotivated that they eat a takeaway meal after work and spend the evening slumped in front of the television. When these kinds of things arise it always means that dehydration is in place and this always means a disconnection of some kind from our higher aspects and therefore from our potential.

2. The Natural Rhythms

The second principle looks at our connectedness to the natural rhythms of the universe. Our bodies work hard to take full advantage of the high energy of the spring and autumn equinoxes as a means of clearing toxicity. It is not uncommon to find with an equinox that a person doesn't resolve their toxicity and this results in an acute episode. Minor symptoms might have been brewing over the preceding months or even years, but when the equinox arrives, major ill health can arise.

Although the equinoxes are times of potential healing through the removal of a high level of toxicity, they are also potentially times when the body can become overwhelmed and be unable to move the story on in a positive direction. This could be seen as an inability to fully resolve an acute illness, so that symptoms drag on for weeks or months afterwards.

We can also look at full and new moons and with women look at how this cycle relates to their menstrual cycle. There is enormous relief and reassurance to be drawn from the realization that we each dance with the energy of the moon. Having an awareness, for instance, that the time of the full moon can be challenging means that if you don't quite feel yourself then, you have no need to worry, because once the full moon has passed you will feel much more yourself again. It is so much easier to endure a challenging situation with pleasure if you know when it is going to end.

When we learn to take notice of our dance with the moon, we can accurately predict challenging times and adjust our energies and lifestyles beforehand so that we are fully ready to embrace the challenge rather than becoming stressed by it. Remember also that every two days the moon brings a focus on a different part of our body.

When you start to make connections with the natural rhythms, it can be a revelation in how it explains so much of your story.

3. The Five Elements

The five elements system is such a beautiful way of looking at connectedness. The seasons, organs and emotions are all interconnected and so we can begin to connect the natural rhythms to how we feel and function.

The autumn equinox falls within the time of the Metal element, which also relates to the skin, colon, lungs and mind. In my practice it is very common for people to come to see me just after the autumn equinox with a severe colon imbalance such as a flare-up of Crohn's disease, colitis or irritable bowel syndrome. There may well have been minor symptoms such as occasional constipation beforehand, but it is so common for the diagnosis of a named disease to take place only after the autumn equinox.

What time of year do you feel most at ease in and which is the most challenging? These times will tell you about which of your organs are strongest and which are weakest and it will also tell you something about your emotions and why you feel the way you do. The five elements are almost limitless in the connections that they can make for us.

4. Hering's Law of Cure

Knowing and applying Hering's Law is a wonderful way of being able to tell whether an illness has been suppressed or released. Remember that Hering's Law states that 'Illness leaves the body from the top to the bottom, from the inside to the outside, from the greater organs to the lesser organs and in the reverse order to which it manifested.' If a person being treated for asthma suddenly became low in energy and depressed, you would know that their story had gone deeper, so the treatment must have been suppressive. If, however, they suddenly manifested an itchy skin which then resolved itself, you would know that they were heading in the right direction because the skin is a much lowlier organ than the lungs.

You can apply Hering's Law to all symptoms of disease and see clearly in which direction you are moving, whether towards or away from health.

5. Acute and Chronic Episodes

It is always good to highlight both acute and chronic episodes within your story. Everyone is born with a certain amount of toxicity passed down to them from their parents. During childhood and the teenage years, acute episodes are created by the body in order to release this toxicity. These will often occur around the equinoxes. When managed correctly, acute illnesses can be keys to unlocking hidden potential, but when suppressed they can further reduce potential.

In really deep stories such as ME, it is quite common to see within a person's story a time when there was an acceleration of acute illnesses as the body tried to release toxicity. Then, because the body became too tired to be able to raise the energy needed to bring about an acute episode, the acute illnesses stopped. The person appeared to have improved in health, with coughs, colds and the 'flu becoming distant memories, but this actually meant that the body's chronic load had increased and the dis-ease had gone deeper.

6. Body Temperature

As people become more toxic, there is always a reduction in body temperature. Likewise, a course of antibiotics will bring about a loss of heat from the body. A lower body temperature means that the energy needed to raise the temperature to the level of a flamboyant fever is too great and so people become less capable of manifesting acute illnesses. In very deep stories such as with ME and AIDS, there is always a lower than normal body temperature. It is also not unusual to find a drop in temperature after the administration of a lot of vaccines. Fortunately we have techniques that can raise the body temperature and recreate the heat needed to burn off toxicity.

7. Body pH

Changes in body pH are usually quite easy to spot. They often manifest as achiness or headaches, both of which are signs that the pH of the blood has fallen. This is usually due to a lack of alkalizing foods or alkalizing (relaxing) activities, but can be equally caused by thinking too many acidic thoughts. Our thoughts and emotions have a particularly strong influence on our body pH. The more stressed we are, the more dehydrated we will be and therefore the more acidic we will be.

8. Blood Sugar

Blood sugar levels are intrinsically linked to energy levels, so any drop in energy will mean that blood sugar levels have become unstable. Remember that low blood sugar can be described as an inability to hold calcium levels correctly in the blood, and this relates back to our day/night exchange. When we are dehydrated, the cell membrane builds up a cholesterol layer which prevents the full flow of sodium and calcium out of the cell during the night. This situation not only affects calcium levels in the blood but also has a knock-on effect on all the factors in our test tube.

A drop in body temperature, a drop in pH, an inability to create acute illness and the stress of both lifestyle and a poor diet will all adversely affect blood sugar levels. Situations where people binge on foods or have massive energy drops during the day with accompanying insatiable hunger are signs of extreme blood sugar problems.

9. The Tubercular Taint

The tubercular taint can be seen in people born with a strong predisposition inherited from their ancestral line. In this situation certain metabolic pathways such as the processing of essential fatty acids are impaired. It is strongly linked to the inability to keep calcium in the right place, so also relates back to blood sugar. It can most easily be seen in the ancestry when one or more ancestors have had tuberculosis that has not been treated correctly and so the person is born with an inherited inability to hold calcium levels correctly within the body.

10. Pasteur/Béchamp

It is interesting to look at your story from the differing perspectives of Pasteur and Béchamp. The Pasteur point of view is that illness comes from an outside invasion and needs to be suppressed or killed. It takes responsibility away from the individual and places it with institutions such as the medical and pharmaceutical industries. It is a viewpoint that creates victims of disease and offers nothing in the way of truly healing solutions. Béchamp, on the other hand, saw that it is the soil and being of each of us that decides our health. Looking at your own case history, you can see how the application of allopathic medicine gradually sends your story deeper and deeper.

11. Light and the Endocrine System

A person's ability to hold and create light is reflected clearly in the functioning of their endocrine system.

Adrenal fatigue, PMT, blood sugar problems, immune weakness and an underactive thyroid are all signs of a weakness in the light-holding ability of a person.

Remember that Hering's Law tells us that an endocrine imbalance will rise from the bottom up, starting with the adrenals. If a person has an endocrine imbalance up to the level of the pituitary, they are likely to feel very cut off from who they really are and to be in the dark about how to find healing. When someone in this situation starts to make connections, you see them literally become more radiant as their path to healing begins to shine before them.

12. 'Never Been Well Since...'

If you have never been well since a particular time, it is often an indicator of a transition not fully accomplished and is highly significant. If, for instance, you had a sore throat that was repeatedly suppressed with antibiotics and you have never been well since, it is a sign that resolution of toxicity in the throat and lymphatic system has not taken place. This resolution will need to unfold at some point during the healing process.

13. Major Transitions

There are several major transitions that take place during a person's life and if a situation of deep stress occurs at those times, it can have a significant effect for many years.

The first transition is conception, where the egg migrates to its correct place. For this to occur it is vital that the electrical charge in and around the womb is correct. An ectopic pregnancy, where the egg develops outside the womb, is caused by the wrong charge in and around the womb.

The next transition is birth. A baby presenting feet first is a lesser sign of the charge in the womb not being correct.

There are three important transitions that need to take place within the first two years of life. When a baby is in the womb, sodium is dominant over potassium within the developing child. This remains so for the first six months after birth, but after this it is important for health that potassium is introduced. Normally at about six months a mother starts introducing vegetables and hence potassium to her baby. By the age of two, the potassium levels need to exceed the sodium levels and in a female child these also need to be slightly higher than in a male child. This is a transition that more and more children are failing to make correctly these days, especially with such high sodium levels in the modern diet.

The second transition relates to the essential fatty acid requirements of a developing child. When a baby is born, its small intestine is porous. In our look at the five elements we saw that the small intestine is regarded as the 'great separator' of the pure from the impure. By the age of two, the small intestine should cease to be porous but the child's ability to do this is totally dependent upon the essential fatty acids it received from its mother both in the womb and through the breast milk. When a mother herself is very deficient in essential fatty acids, the small intestine of her child can remain porous beyond the age of two. Psoriasis and leaky gut syndrome are both signs of a porous small intestine.

The third transition relates to the levels of copper and zinc within the baby. At the end of the pregnancy, copper levels rise dramatically in order to facilitate the contractions of labour. When copper becomes dominant, zinc levels drop accordingly and this low zinc level is passed on to the baby. Low zinc levels can cause many health problems, so it is vital for the baby's health that they rise again after birth. Fortunately nature provides a wonderful way in which to redress this imbalance. The placenta is very rich in zinc and when a mother eats her placenta, the zinc is passed via the colostrum to the baby to redress this imbalance. Humans are the only animals that do not eat the placenta after birth and an important transition is interrupted as a result. Copper levels remain high and this is linked to dependency. The baby has high copper levels in the womb because it is totally dependent upon its mother, but by the age of two zinc levels should have risen so that the child can begin to find its independence.

Puberty is another transition that makes many demands on the body. The production of sexual hormones at this time makes strong demands on the body for zinc. If the body is low in zinc anyway, copper will become very dominant at this time and we can see this manifesting as co-dependent, addictive behaviour during puberty. The contraceptive pill also increases copper levels, which can increase the co-dependent behaviour if it is given soon after puberty to relieve menstrual problems.

In women, pregnancy, giving birth and the menopause

are also important transitions, each of which needs to be navigated with the skill of connectedness.

Our final transition is death. For many people the thought of it evokes fear, but when someone is healthy and connected, death is just another doorway to walk through with joy.

CHAPTER 8

THE THREE STAGES
OF TREATMENT

The three stages of treatment is a pattern of working with people that seeks to avoid adding any extra stress to the body. When someone is particularly unwell, they will often have a lot of different symptoms. Some alternative therapists would look to treat all of these symptoms with a barrage of supplements, herbs or remedies, but that has the potential to just add further stress and becomes no different from allopathic treatment. It is not *what* we use that is most important, but *how* we use it.

The three stages of treatment aim to return integrity to a person in the reverse order from how it was lost. It is a process of gently opening up the energetic pathways within the body so that the person can connect to their inner wisdom. It is a way of empowering them and giving them permission to listen to how they feel, because the answers are only to be found within. You know how to heal yourself. If you feel that you do not know, it is only because the message has become obscured by toxicity. Gently allow the body to let go of what is no longer needed and healing must follow.

You can see that this is really the complete opposite of the approach adopted by so many doctors and alternative practitioners, who treat symptoms and prescribe in an allopathic way. If I meet a person who has parasites, I would not be looking to give them a potion to kill those parasites. Surely parasites are part of this amazing universe and have as much right to life as you and I? Isn't killing them going against natural law? The three stages are designed to change the conditions in the test tube of the host so as to create an environment that is not conducive to parasites. Then the parasites will naturally leave the body in search of a better home. This is working in partnership with nature rather than trying to override her perfect patterns and rhythms. We must remember that it is the responsibility of each individual to restore balance and harmony to their own vehicle rather than putting the blame on an outside invader or pathogen.

Woven throughout the three stages is an intent to open a person up to all of the natural rhythms. In order to be in harmony with life, our bodies are set up to respond to these rhythms. Our cells dance with the sun and the moon as they go through their 24-hour cycle of metabolizing and cleansing, our organs dance to the tune of the unfolding day, and the energies and light flowing through each of us ebb and flow in time with the seasons. Certain times of year, such as the equinoxes, provide us with extra energy for cleansing, but we need to be able to respond to these special times if we are to take advantage of this energy.

When you gently open a person up in this way and remind them of who they really are, you begin to see a dramatic increase in human potential. Where once a disease was labelled as incurable, now there is the vision of a path back to health. Where life was dull and unfulfilling, now there is a growing passion to discover just how wonderful and adventurous life can become. The most exciting journey you will ever take is the one to discover who you really are and just how many amazing things you are capable of.

If we want to release toxicity, we need to gently support the routes of elimination that exist within the body. In the next chapter I will talk about some simple but amazing techniques that you can use to help this process. If we want healing to be a stress-free process of forever increasing opening, it is vital that we match the push and pull of toxicity within the body so that the speed of release of toxicity from the cell is matched by the speed of elimination from the body. What we do not want to do is to pull toxicity out of one place in the body and then push it into another. This might appear to cure some symptoms but would actually create another disease. We each need to be personally vigilant and aware of this movement.

True healing requires us to open up blocked pathways within the body in the reverse order in which they closed.

We will look to switch off the dehydration alert mechanically to open the cells, then to restore the central nervous system, which is where all the fear is held, and to balance the endocrine system. Then we will look at the balance of our four main electrolytes and their relationship to the overall charge. When the charge is correct, the hydration is correct. When the hydration is correct, we can fully utilize light and be deeply in touch with all of the natural rhythms.

Stage One
The Case History

Stage One begins with taking the case history. The person being treated is in their own space, telling their own story in chronological order. I take note of how episodes of illness have been treated in the past and also look at the health of the ancestors back at least as far as the grandparents. Questions are asked about diet, lifestyle, current medication and/or supplements and any other relevant information.

This is followed by the most important aspect of Stage One: the interpretation. Handing back to a person the understanding of how their dis-ease manifested is so important in enabling them to move on. When a case history is properly interpreted, they suddenly see the connectedness of their symptoms. This is in stark contrast to the reductionist approach of treating those symptoms individually. This gives them a powerful insight into the amazing integrity of their body and immediately their level of fear will begin to drop. As soon as fear begins to subside, hydration will automatically start to improve, and this is before any suggestions have been made regarding what to eat and drink and what supplements might be useful.

The moment fear reduces there is also an increase in personal power and this results in an energetic change within the individual. This energetic change is so important because it enables a person to leave a consultation feeling brighter, lighter and enthusiastic about their unfolding journey back to health. The purpose of the interpretation is to empower the person and to *energetically* switch off the dehydration alert within them.

So in Stage One we begin to change the conditions in the test tube whilst being very aware, having looked at the case history, of the predispositions that the individual was born with. Depending on the predispositions, it becomes clear how much we need to support them in their process of change and empowerment.

Diet and Fluids

Next we look at diet and fluids, because with these we can *mechanically* switch off the dehydration alert. It takes time to fundamentally change the body biochemistry and we address this in Stages Two and Three, but with the correct diet, fluids and techniques you can dramatically change the way a person feels.

All food holds a vibration and each food therefore will offer a vibrational challenge to our bodies. This vibration can be changed depending upon how the food is grown, harvested and prepared for eating. It might be obvious that there will be a difference in the quality of a chicken depending on whether it is produced by intensive farming or natural and organic means, but the same is true of all foods. Just because oils, meats and vegetables are made to look attractive in many modern supermarkets does not mean that they necessarily provide good nutrition. When you add an array of chemicals to foods, such as pesticides, fungicides and preservatives, you add many unnatural vibrations into that food, and whatever vibrations you take in through your mouth have to be interpreted by your body.

Similarly, fluids are vital if we are to rehydrate the body, but they must be the correct fluids, as not all liquids are hydrating. Caffeinated drinks, including black tea and coffee, alcohol, sweetened soft drinks and drinks containing colourings and aspartame, all have a diuretic effect on the body, effectively increasing dehydration, so these are all gradually removed from the diet and replaced with clean water. Once this changeover has taken place I recommend drinking between two and two and a half litres of water at body temperature each day, but never more than one litre in any given hour.

Sugar creates a loss of magnesium and is also drying, so this is removed also.

Next I look at carbohydrates, especially grains. There is a hierarchy of challenge with grains, meaning some grains are easier to digest than others. The most challenging of the grains is wheat, followed by rye and then oats and barley. These four glutinous grains are all acid forming and can present a strong challenge to anyone who is overly acidic or dehydrated. At the lower end of the scale are short-grain brown rice and millet. Both these are considered to be gluten-free grains. Depending upon the person's story, we might need to remove wheat from the diet, gluten from the diet or even initially remove all grains. The Chinese regard short-grain brown rice as 'the food of the colon' and it is an ideal food to help hydration as long as the person is able to digest it.

When I first began treating people I found it to be quite common to need to remove wheat from the diet. Later on in my work it became more common to need to remove all the gluten grains. Today I find many more people who initially cannot tolerate any grains. In these cases quinoa, which is actually a seed rather than a grain, becomes a very useful alternative.

The next category I look at is vegetables and juices. Vegetables should account for at least 50 per cent of two of the meals during the day and it is best to eat them in a seasonal way. This means not only looking at which vegetables grow in a particular season but also deciding whether they should be predominantly cooked or raw. If blood sugar is implicated, it is often necessary to concentrate more on leafy vegetables than the sweeter root vegetables until the blood sugar remains consistently stable.

Juicing can be very valuable as it helps to promote cleansing within the body, but one needs to be cautious when juicing fruit, as this can be overly cleansing and sweet, which might be too challenging.

Fruit is best eaten in a seasonal manner, meaning that in a temperate climate fresh fruit would only be consumed during the summer and during the winter dried fruit would be used.

Next I look at proteins. Proteins can be acid forming, but they are also good stabilizers of blood sugar, so often need to be included in meals, especially if blood sugar levels are unstable. In terms of meat, red meats are the most acid forming and are usually avoided, while white meats such as chicken are much less challenging. Fish and eggs are both excellent sources of animal protein, but vegetarian forms of protein include pulses, nuts, seeds and bee pollen. Whenever meat and fish are eaten, one can balance out their acid-forming properties by adding plenty of alkalizing leafy green vegetables to the meal. Eggs can be a problem for some people who suffer from asthma, but for most people they are an excellent source of protein and can be eaten every day if desired.

Some people find pulses difficult to digest, but they are made much more digestible if soaked overnight and even more so if they are left until they just start to sprout. Nuts, seeds and pulses are actually vegetables in a dormant form, so it is best to always soak them before eating as this makes them more digestible. Soaked nuts and seeds are excellent when made into milks or butters. Seeds that have just begun sprouting can be used for protein, but once the sprout has fully formed the seed changes from a protein to a vegetable. One should also note that for pulses to count as a complete protein, they must be mixed with a type of grain or with sesame seeds. A complete protein is one that has the full range of amino acids present in the stomach at the same time.

The next category of foods is dairy produce. In the West most dairy produce is pasteurized and much of it is also homogenized. Both of these processes change what is a natural product into one that is both unnatural and of little nutritional value. Furthermore, by the age of two we lose the enzymes required to break down and utilize milk, because that is normally the end of the breastfeeding phase.

Yoghurt has been partially digested by the bacteria present within it and so presents much less of a challenge. When it is made from a less processed milk such as goat's milk it is even less challenging.

Cheese can be very challenging because most of it is pasteurized and has had salt added to it in order to harden it. Consuming foods high in sodium presents a strong challenge to anyone who is dehydrated.

Generally, dairy produce, with the exception of yoghurt, butter and ghee, presents too high a challenge for the body to digest and would be best replaced by seed and nut milks. Also, dairy products have a tendency to unbalance the electrolytes (sodium, calcium, potassium and magnesium) and are mucous forming, meaning that they tend to thicken and thus reduce the flow of lymph.

Perhaps the least understood of all the main food groups are the fats and oils, especially when it comes to cooking with them. Contrary to popular belief, we should not be cooking with mono- and poly-unsaturated fats such as olive oil and vegetable oils because they become seriously damaged when exposed to heat. It is so important for our health to not eat damaged fats, including trans fats and hydrogenated fats, because they dramatically reduce the porosity of our cell membranes. When this happens it interrupts all of the natural rhythms and functioning within our body tissue. Virgin olive oil and other cold-pressed vegetable oils should only be added to food after it has been cooked. The safest oils for cooking are actually the saturated fats, because they are chemically very stable even when exposed to heat, so butter, butter ghee and coconut oil are the best to use for cooking.

Sample Diets for Stage One

Everyone is unique and therefore the dietary recommendations for each person will also be unique, but there are some general guidelines we can use when treating different levels of toxicity and illness. When creating a diet, we need to use foods that present the minimum challenge to the body. This means using foods in their natural state and avoiding all artificial additives, colourings and preservatives. In doing this we can be sure that the body will recognize the food and be able to process it with the minimum of effort, thus creating extra energy that can be focused upon healing. Sugar, aspartame and other artificial sweeteners must be avoided, likewise table salt.

In each of the following diets we are going to address each of the different categories of food as mentioned above.

In all the following diets fluids should be addressed first. This means avoiding drinks containing caffeine and replacing them with herbal (not fruit) teas or grain coffees, avoiding alcohol and sugary drinks, and consuming two to two and a half litres of clean water at body temperature every day.

GUIDELINES FOR A GENERAL MAINTENANCE DIET

Fresh Vegetables	Eat two meals during the day consisting of 50 per cent fresh vegetables. Some should be cooked and some should be raw (depending on the season). Drink half a pint (a quarter of a litre) of freshly pressed vegetable juice (consumed within 20 minutes of making) daily.
Fruit	Eat two pieces of fruit daily. Try to be seasonal in your choices.
Proteins (vegetarians and vegans will need to replace animal proteins with vegetable protein)	Eat white meat (twice a week), fish (twice a week, one being oily fish), red meat (once a week), eggs (three days a week) and on two days a week avoid all animal proteins (use vegetable proteins instead, e.g. pulses).
Fats	For cooking, use butter ghee, butter or coconut oil. All other oils should be added after cooking. Avoid hydrogenated and trans-fatty acids. Ideal dressings include olive oil, walnut oil, pumpkin seed oil and argon oil.
Carbohydrates	Potatoes should be restricted to once a week (belladonna family). Sweet potatoes, cassava, quinoa, maize and buckwheat are good carbo-hydrate sources.
Grains	Unrefined grains should be used. Try to choose an alternative to wheat whenever possible, e.g. rye bread. Short-grain brown rice is an ideal grain for the maintenance of health.

GUIDELINES FOR AN ALKALIZING DIET

Fresh Vegetables	Eat two meals during the day consisting of 70 per cent fresh vegetables. Some should be cooked and some should be raw (depending on the season). Drink half a pint (a quarter of a litre) of freshly pressed vegetable juice (consumed within 20 minutes of making) daily.
Fruit	Eat two pieces of fruit daily. Try to be seasonal in your choices. No citrus.
Proteins (vegetarians and vegans will need to replace animal proteins with vegetable protein)	Eat fish (three times a week, one being oily fish) and on four days a week avoid all animal proteins (use vegetable proteins instead, e.g. pulses).
Dairy (if no allergy is present)	Try to use as little as possible and choose unhomogenized and organic. Goat's yoghurt would be acceptable.
Fats	For cooking, use butter ghee, butter or coconut oil. All other oils should be added after cooking. Avoid hydrogenated and trans-fatty acids. Ideal dressings include olive oil, walnut oil, pumpkin seed oil and argon oil.
Carbohydrates	Use sweet potatoes or quinoa.
Grains	Use short-grain brown rice (twice daily).

GUIDELINES FOR A BLOOD SUGAR STABILIZING DIET

Fresh Vegetables	Eat two meals during the day consisting of 50 per cent fresh vegetables. Some should be cooked and some should be raw (depending on the season). Avoid using too many root vegetables due to their sweetness. Drink half a pint (a quarter of a litre) of freshly pressed vegetable juice (consumed within 20 minutes of making) daily. Avoid using too many root vegetables due to their sweetness.
Fruit	Avoid.
Proteins (vegetarians and vegans will need to replace animal proteins with vegetable protein)	Eat animal protein at breakfast and possibly in a second meal during the day. Use vegetable protein for the third meal. Try to eat one hour before going to bed.
Dairy (if no allergy is present)	Try to use as little as possible and choose unhomogenized and organic. Goat's yoghurt would be acceptable.
Fats	For cooking, use butter ghee, butter or coconut oil. All other oils should be added after cooking. Avoid hydrogenated and trans-fatty acids. Ideal dressings include olive oil, walnut oil, pumpkin seed oil and argon oil.
Carbohydrates	Use quinoa.
Grains	Use short-grain brown rice.

*When tackling low blood sugar, eating little and often helps initially.

GUIDELINES FOR A GLUTEN-FREE DIET

Fresh Vegetables	Eat two meals during the day consisting of 50 per cent fresh vegetables. Some should be cooked and some should be raw (depending on the season). Drink half a pint (a quarter of a litre) of freshly pressed vegetable juice (consumed within 20 minutes of making) daily.
Fruit	Eat two pieces of fruit daily. Try to be seasonal in your choices.
Proteins (vegetarians and vegans will need to replace animal proteins with vegetable protein)	Eat white meat (twice a week), fish (twice a week, one being oily fish), red meat (once a week), eggs (three days a week) and on two days a week avoid all animal proteins (use vegetable proteins instead, e.g. pulses).
Dairy (if no allergy is present)	Try to use as little as possible and choose unhomogenized and organic. Goat's yoghurt would be acceptable.
Fats	For cooking, use butter ghee, butter or coconut oil. All other oils should be added after cooking. Avoid hydrogenated and trans-fatty acids. Ideal dressings include olive oil, walnut oil, pumpkin seed oil and argon oil.
Carbohydrates	Potatoes should be restricted to once a week (belladonna family). Sweet potatoes, cassava, quinoa, maize and buckwheat are good carbohydrate sources.
Grains	Only short-grain brown rice or millet should be used.

GUIDELINES TO BREAK AN ADDICTIVE-EATING DIET

Fresh Vegetables	Eat three meals during the day consisting of 60 per cent fresh vegetables. Some should be cooked and some should be raw (depending on the season). Avoid using too many root vegetables due to their sweetness. Drink half a pint (a quarter of a litre) of freshly pressed vegetable juice (consumed within 20 minutes of making) daily.
Fruit	Avoid.
Proteins (vegetarians and vegans will need to replace animal proteins with vegetable protein)	Use animal protein for two meals a day and vegetable protein (e.g. tofu) for the third meal. Initially, animal protein may be required for all three meals in the day to stabilise blood sugar.
Dairy (if no allergy is present)	Try to use as little as possible and choose unhomogenized and organic. Goat's yoghurt would be acceptable.
Fats	For cooking, use butter ghee, butter or coconut oil. All other oils should be added after cooking. Avoid hydrogenated and trans-fatty acids. Ideal dressings include olive oil, walnut oil, pumpkin seed oil and argon oil.
Carbohydrates	Avoid all carbohydrates, although quinoa may be acceptable.
Grains	Avoid all grains.

Food Combining

A very effective way to lessen the pressure on a weakened digestive system is to use food combining. This is particularly useful for cases of bloating or to combat acidity. Food combining recognizes the fact that proteins and carbohydrates have differing pH requirements within the stomach. By separating these two groups, the body has fewer mixed messages to deal with, and thus stress on the digestive system is reduced.

The rules of food combining are as follows:

- Never combine animal protein and carbohydrate in any meal.
- Vegetables can be used with either an animal protein or a carbohydrate meal.

- Fruit (other than bananas or sweet pears) can be used with any animal protein meal.
- Bananas and sweet pears can be used with any carbohydrate meal.
- Yoghurt can be used with either an animal protein or a carbohydrate meal.
- Rice and pulses (non-animal protein) can be combined.

A typical meal plan when food combining would be:

- *Breakfast*: Carbohydrate (e.g. toast) and a banana
- *Lunch*: Animal protein (e.g. fish) and vegetables and fruit (except bananas and sweet pears)
- *Dinner*: Carbohydrate (e.g. rice) and vegetables.

Other Useful Tools

Eating a mono meal can be very useful when wanting to release extra energy for healing. A mono meal consists of just one ingredient so that the stomach requires the minimum effort to digest it. A single vegetable soup or a bowl of short-grain brown rice are both examples of such meals. A mono meal in the evening can be very useful for people who have digestive problems at night.

Finally in Stage One are the techniques. These are powerful tools that anyone can use to support the body through its process of healing. These will be fully explained in the next chapter.

So, during Stage One we've gained an understanding of the story, we've taken the stress away and we've switched off the dehydration alert.

Stage Two

In Stage Two we look at supporting the central nervous system and the endocrine system. What we are doing here is beginning to change the biochemistry.

Reassuring the Colon

The most important thing is to maintain a strong message to the colon that it is hydrated, so we start by using linseed tea.

To make linseed tea you take two tablespoons of linseeds and add one litre of clean water. You bring this mixture to the boil, turn off the heat, cover and leave to stand away from the heat for 12 hours or overnight. You then gently simmer the tea for one hour, strain off the seeds and make a tea out of some of the thickened liquid mixed with hot water. This is ideal for giving the colon a strong message of hydration.

The tea can be drunk throughout the day and the remaining thick liquid can be stored in the fridge once it has cooled down, and used for making linseed tea over the next two days.

If you are using a diet which is low in grains, drinking linseed tea half an hour before each meal can be very useful for giving the correct message to the colon. This is particularly useful when following a diet for addictive eating or to balance blood sugar levels.

Essential Fatty Acids

Having reassured the colon, we can then move on to look at essential fatty acids more closely. Fish oils, with their high levels of EPA and DHA, can be very helpful initially, especially because so many people have lost their ability to break down oils. Remember that fish oils are broken-down omega 3 essential fatty acids.

Once the condition of the person has improved, we can move onto flax oil, which is predominantly parent (unbroken-down) omega 3. Flax oil has a ratio of omega 3:6 of 4:1, whereas hemp oil, which some people use as their main source of essential fatty acids, has an omega 3:6 ratio of 1:3. It is much more beneficial to have a higher ratio of omega 3 to omega 6.

All these oils containing essential fatty acids must be taken with some form of protein, because our bodies need the sulphur bonds contained within the amino acids of the proteins to be able to utilize these oils correctly. Bee pollen and Liquid Aminos, which is a savoury liquid, both provide these sulphur bonds. If you can use yoghurt, a nice way to take oils is to mix them into the yoghurt with some lecithin and bee pollen. Oils can also be taken with a meal containing some form of animal protein. Lecithin granules are also taken along with the oils and protein. Lecithin is an emulsifier, meaning that it helps the oils to mix with the water within the body. They are rich in phospholipids and contain a good amount of omega 6 (25 per cent).

Some people find oils and lecithin challenging to take and can suffer from nausea or low energy as a result. There are supplements that can support people if this occurs, but it is not possible within the scope of this book to give further details because every person is unique and there-fore requires a different prescription.

The Endocrine System

After the essential fatty acids, we would go on to look at the endocrine system. The body needs to be able to constantly produce 30 different prostaglandins (tissue hormones) and to do so requires adequate amounts of omega 3 (especially EPA), omega 6, magnesium, zinc and vitamins B3, B6, C and E. This is perhaps where I might look at supplementation, providing the level of hydration had improved to a point where the person was no longer feeling fearful. I use a high-quality multi-vitamin and mineral supplement in such cases. Sometimes it is also useful to look at supporting the thyroid and adrenal glands with appropriate supplementation or herbs, but again this has to be done on a personal basis.

Stage Three
Electrolytes and Trace Minerals

This is where we begin to look at the four main electrolytes: sodium, potassium, calcium and magnesium.

The most important of these to look at in terms of supplementation is magnesium, because it is deficient in most soils and therefore in most vegetables, even organic ones. When supplementing magnesium I find that the citrate form works best. This is because the body makes a lot of citrate, so is less likely to be concerned if a little more is added. I use between 100 and 400mg of elemental magnesium. Magnesium also requires vitamin B6 to work, but this would have been addressed when looking at the endocrine system. All supplements should only be taken for six out of every seven days to allow the body a day of rest from them.

Potassium levels tend to be less of a problem, provided people are consuming plenty of vegetables in their diet.

It is actually very unusual to need to supplement calcium. This is because there is usually a plentiful supply of it in the diet. So often I find that what appears to be a low level of calcium in the body is often actually misplaced calcium that finds its correct place again once the body is hydrated and has enough magnesium.

Sodium is likewise found in plentiful supply in vegetables.

Finally at the end of Stage Three I would look at the levels of trace minerals.

The process of the three stages allows healing to take place gently and sequentially. Throughout the process we are gradually increasing the hydration and gradually changing the pH, temperature and light utilization, and what we find is that parasites or candida overgrowths will leave the body if the conditions in the test tube have changed in this way.

The most important parts of the process are Stage One and the first part of Stage Two, addressing fluids, diet and oils, because once a person is more hydrated and able to hold light around their cell membranes, they become much more connected to their inner wisdom. Through this reconnection, they begin to attract the solutions they need to bring their healing process to its full potential.

Remember that the body never works against us and that fear is the only thing that stops us doing what we feel we want to do. When you are fully hydrated, all fears subside and freedom moves from a possibility to a certainty. This is not only freedom from dis-ease but also freedom to dream and then to fulfil those dreams.

CHAPTER 9

THE MAGIC OF TECHNIQUES

In this chapter I want to introduce you to a range of simple yet powerful techniques. For me they form the most important part of my practice and I have, over the years, found them to be uniquely effective.

If we are asking the body to become well, this requires a fair amount of energy in order to bring about the necessary movement for cleansing, balancing and purification. Usually this energy comes from the body itself, but if someone is ill or overtired, their ability to bring forth extra energy is often impaired. This is where techniques can be extremely useful.

With techniques, we are either wanting to create movement in stagnant areas, or we are wanting to bring heat to cold areas, or we are just wanting to bring more energy to a particular area where energy is very low. Using careful selection and a holistic understanding, we can employ techniques to provide that much-needed energy to start creating movement. Even more importantly, the following techniques can be utilized to ensure that any stagnation or toxicity which starts to be released continues to move all of the way out of the body.

The techniques vary greatly, as each targets a particular area of the body or supports a particular process. However, they all have a common goal: to help the body achieve balance in areas where it is struggling. They enable us to access any part of the body and offer it some assistance.

When employing techniques, it is important to be sympathetic to what you are asking the body to do. It is all too easy, with over-enthusiasm, to make too many changes without considering what the consequences of those changes might be. When the body is not healthy, it is basically under-functioning and therefore all of its systems are in some way impaired. To start shifting excessive amounts of stagnation or toxicity and to expect these impaired systems to cope with this extra workload on their own is unrealistic. Patience is required if you want to bring your body back to health. You must endeavour to release a manageable amount of toxicity when you begin changing your diet and lifestyle. Also, it is important to ensure that the toxicity moves through all of the levels of detoxification and out of the body. This can be managed with the aid of techniques. Once you have released the initial toxicity from the body and it is in a slightly improved state of health, you can then re-evaluate the situation and perhaps employ further treatment and managed elimination. This is where listening to your body becomes vitally important. It needs to be gradually returned to balance rather than overloaded with mobilized toxicity.

With this in mind, let us look again at the process of detoxification and how we can support it.

How Does the Body Detoxify?

The body has a set process for detoxifying and all of the stages of that process need to be functioning well for health to be returned and maintained.

Remember that in a healthy body toxins are removed automatically using the following route:

1. Toxicity is released at a cellular level into the lymphatic system (some toxins leave the lymph and are released from the body via the skin and lungs).
2. The toxic lymph then drains into the blood (some of the toxins leave the blood and are released from the body via the skin and lungs).
3. The blood passes through the liver and the liver filters out the toxins.
4. The liver excretes the toxic bile into the bowel.
5. From the bowel the toxins are excreted from the body.

What Happens If Detoxification Is Impaired?

In a body where detoxification is impaired, toxicity can get blocked at any of the above stages. For example, the toxicity released from the cell can stagnate in the lymph. If this toxicity is allowed to stagnate for a long time, the body will begin to show signs of illness such as swollen glands or a sore throat. These symptoms arise as the body attempts to move the stagnation onwards. It might even create a fever to thin and move the lymph. In this example you can offer the lymphatic system some assistance by employing techniques. If you can help to move this stagnation from the lymph, the body can then attempt to finish the process and excrete the toxins.

To take another example, if the liver becomes overloaded with toxicity, the toxins will back up in the blood, and if the bowel is sluggish, the whole system of detoxification grinds to a halt. In order for the liver to release its toxic bile freely into the bowel, the bowel needs to be evacuating effectively. You can begin to see just how important it is for our health and wellbeing that this primary route of elimination is open and working freely. If this is not occurring, there are some techniques in this chapter to rectify the situation.

In reality, in the first example, it would not be possible to have stagnation in only the lymphatic system. There would also have to be significant stagnation within the liver and the blood to cause the kind of symptoms described.

Due to its important role as the main internal organ of elimination, the liver is normally the first place to show congestion when the body is trying to heal and rebalance. If it begins to struggle with its role of detoxifying the blood, the level of toxicity within the blood begins to rise. If this situation is left unsupported, the blood system will struggle to receive and cleanse the lymph effectively. The lymph will therefore become thicker as its own level of toxicity begins to rise. If this situation is also left unattended, the cell will begin to have trouble releasing into the lymph system and this will cause cellular congestion.

In my experience, no matter which stage of the elimination process appears to be struggling, it is the liver that always needs supporting first. When you support the liver with techniques you improve its efficiency during the detoxification process. Once the liver is coping, you can then return to the original area of congestion and apply the appropriate techniques to create movement. Then the liver will usually require further support to ensure that it can deal with the extra toxicity as it is released.

The real art in using these techniques is in keeping the speed of elimination at an even rate throughout all of the systems from the cell to the outside of the body. If this is achieved, the detoxification and healing process will be comfortable and continually empowering. It will also ensure that no areas of the body are left unsupported. However, this requires you to take full responsibility for yourself and how you feel. For me, techniques are about empowering the individual to take personal responsibility for their healing and to give them the tools to make health a reality. So let us explore these techniques.

Skin Brushing

The skin is the largest organ of elimination; this makes it a very important organ to work on when supporting the body's natural healing process. The purpose of skin brushing is to first remove the scurf layer (the uppermost layer of skin), which holds a certain amount of acidity and toxicity. To brush this layer away makes a whole new surface area available through which to excrete toxins. Brushing the skin also promotes movement within the lymphatic system and thus helps to prevent stagnation and the thickening of the lymph. Thickening of the lymph often happens when the body performs a cleansing process. This is because when the body releases toxicity the lymphatic system has to work hard to move the toxicity to the blood, but without the benefit of a pump (unlike the circulatory system with the heart).

Skin brushing can benefit everyone on a daily basis because it can help to move both toxins and mucous through the body to be released. Excess toxicity and mucous in the lymphatic system can easily stagnate if not kept freely moving.

If you are constipated, it is best to avoid skin brushing, as it will create more material needing to be excreted via the bowel. In this case it would be best to support the bowel first with other techniques.

To skin brush you need a moderately stiff brush. A back brush with a handle is ideal, as it makes reaching all of the body very simple. You can purchase brushes especially designed for skin brushing from many health stores and internet health sites. Keep the brush just for skin brushing. It is best not to wet it, as it will lose its effectiveness.

Skin brushing is applied to dry skin to ensure the scurf layer is easily removed. It is appropriate to do it in the morning or the evening. The movement of the brushing is always towards the heart, as this is where the lymph enters the bloodstream. Do not apply skin brushing to varicose veins, painful rashes or open wounds.

Instructions:

1. Start brushing with gentle but brisk strokes on the top of the right foot and work your way up the entire right leg (front and back). The brush strokes should be felt but should not be painful.
2. Brush on top of the left foot and work your way up the entire left leg.
3. Brush the front and then the back torso upwards towards the heart.
4. Brush the right hand and work your way up the entire right arm up to the shoulder.
5. Brush the left hand and work your way up the entire left arm up to the shoulder.
6. Brush from the neck down to the heart on first the back and then the front torso. Do not brush the face or head.

Skin brushing can have a similar effect to taking exercise. It can make you feel more refreshed and alert, due to the movement it creates within your body. It can help take away that tired feeling that some people experience first thing in the morning or after work in the evening. It is particularly helpful in cases of ME when a person is feeling more tired in the morning than before they went to bed, due to the night-time stagnation of their system. These people are usually too ill to take exercise and so skin brushing can greatly help to get things moving.

Hot and Cold Showering

This technique helps to create movement within the circulatory system, which in turn has a knock-on effect on the lymphatic system. The lymphatic system travels around the body in very close proximity to the blood circulatory system and so anything that speeds up circulation will also help to create movement within the lymph.

Hot and cold showering magnifies the effect of skin brushing, so a beautiful sequence is to do skin brushing first and to follow this by hot and cold showering.

When the body is subjected to heat (e.g. a hot shower), the blood moves in greater volume to the surface of the body (i.e. the skin). This enables the body to lose heat more readily to ensure an even temperature is maintained within the body's vital organs. When the blood moves to the surface, the lymph will follow.

When you subject the body to cold (e.g. a cold shower), the blood moves in greater volume to the inner body. This enables the body to keep the inner vital organs warm and ensure that a balanced temperature is maintained at all times. When the blood moves to the inner body, once again the lymph will follow.

This means that by simply warming and then cooling the body, we can increase the activity within the circulatory system. In doing this we also increase movement within the lymphatic system.

Hot and cold showers can be taken at any time of the

day, but are especially useful first thing in the morning (after skin brushing). This can help the body to begin shifting any stagnation that has arisen overnight. The skin brushing starts to create movement within the lymph and a hot and cold shower afterwards can capitalize on this and provide increased power for accelerated movement.

NB It is very important that this technique is not applied in such a way as to bring stress or shock to the body. Some people are unable to cope with vast differences in temperature, especially those who are pregnant or suffer from a heart condition or high blood pressure. Set the temperatures at levels which suit you and then slowly increase the differential over time.

Instructions:

1. Have a wash in a normal warm shower.
2. Turn the temperature gauge to cool or cold (depending on your level of tolerance) and remain in the shower until your body feels cool or cold.
3. Turn the gauge back to warm or hot (again depending on your level of tolerance) and remain in the shower until your body feels warm again.
4. Repeat this process twice (i.e. three times in total) and be sure to finish on a cool or cold shower.

Hot and cold showers have a similar effect to skin brushing but normally to a greater degree. They can make you feel refreshed and alert, as if you have just kick-started your system into action. They can be particularly useful in situations where people experience sore throats and where the lymph glands in the neck begin to swell. If this situation is left unsupported, the body will want to create a fever to heat the body, thus thinning the lymph and accelerating movement.

If a person is very low in body energy, hot and cold showering can be invaluable, as it is able to supply energy to the body to get the system started and begin to move the stagnation.

Hot and Cold Tubbing

This technique is a deeper and more extreme version of hot and cold showering and therefore has the potential to create a great deal of change within a person, especially in situations of extreme stagnation. When the body is heated up to create a temperature, it has the following effects:

- It helps to melt the cholesterol layer surrounding the cell that hinders the elimination of toxins from the cell in a situation of dehydration alert. Once this layer has been melted, the toxins are able to leave the cell and enter the lymphatic system for removal.
- It heats up the lymphatic system, making the lymph thinner and more fluid. This allows the lymphatic system to better cope with the increased workload created by the cellular release of toxicity and to move the toxins further out of the system ready for excretion.
- It makes the blood move to the surface of the body, and this, as in the previous technique, promotes further movement within the lymphatic system to aid proper elimination.

- It opens the pores, enabling further elimination through the skin itself.

When the body is cooled down, it has the following effects:

- The body produces latent heat from deep within to warm itself and counteract the cold conditions. This movement of heat from within to without produces increased energy for elimination.

As this technique is so powerful at bringing about deep change within a person, it needs to be used with care and at the correct time. It is a wonderful way to promote elimination, but you must be sure that in doing it you do not overload the system, causing a new set of problems. It is not wise to use this technique without having already made significant changes to help open up the routes of elimination.

This technique is invaluable in cases where the cells are overly protected by cholesterol and have thus lost their ability to fully release toxins into the lymphatic system. It is also most useful in situations where the body temperature is very low due to high levels of toxicity and dehydration and when the body is showing signs of viral activity. It can also be used by people who are not showing any great symptoms but simply want to help the body flush out toxins. It is a wonderful way to cleanse the cells and help the body reach a state where it can complete its detoxification cycles with ease.

This technique is ideally used before bed so that you can sleep through the night and allow the body to process the released toxicity. It is ideal to use if your body has lost its ability to naturally produce a fever.

NB Do not use this technique where there is a risk of haemorrhaging, high blood pressure or in pregnancy. Also avoid just after eating, as this may cause nausea.

To apply this technique you need:

- a normal household bath
- a body thermometer
- a small towel
- a hot water bottle (to help warm the body at the end of the technique)
- another person to help oversee the technique and to provide support if required.

Instructions:

1. Lie in a bath at a normal bath temperature.
2. Apply a cool wet towel to your head to ensure that it does not get too hot.
3. Add hot water to the bath at a gradual rate to begin raising the body temperature. Continue with this process until either the temperature has reached 102°F (38.9°C) or, prior to achieving that temperature, you feel that you are as hot as you are able to tolerate. (NB It is not safe to raise the body temperature to more than 102°F unless you are in a supervised clinical

environment.) Be sure to monitor your body temperature throughout by placing the thermometer in your mouth and to keep your head cool.

4. When you feel that you have had enough time in the hot water (every person's limits are different) or you have managed to maintain your body temperature at 102°F for 20 minutes, start to add cold water to the bath. This will gradually start to bring the body temperature down.

5. Take the bath temperature down to a cold but manageable level and lie in it until your body is feeling cold.

6. Once this state has been reached, get out of the bath. You can either dry yourself by rubbing yourself with your bare hands to create friction or you can dry yourself with a towel. Then go to bed with a hot water bottle. Once in bed your body will start to produce heat in order to return its temperature to normal. Keep checking your temperature with the thermometer to ensure that it is increasing at a steady rate. Warm socks and hats can be used if required.

Hot and cold tubbing can produce differing effects depending upon the individual. Often people feel very relaxed and tired afterwards, but some can feel invigorated and ready for action. Occasionally a temporary feeling of nausea (due to bile release) or light-headedness (due to a reduction in blood pressure) can occur.

Some of the most exciting work done with this technique was performed by Douglas Lewis. As mentioned earlier, he observed that the HIV virus was only able to sustain itself in low body temperatures and reasoned that if you heated the body up to provide an artificial fever, changes would occur which would make it non-viable for the virus. He found that the symptoms were gradually cured.

Hot Tub, Cold Wrap

This technique is the same as the previous technique but the cold tubbing section is replaced by a cold damp wrap. This works in the same way as cold tubbing, but with the following advantages:

- It encourages the movement of latent heat from a deeper level within the body. This is because the body has not only to return its own temperature to normal, but also to work much harder in order to dry and warm the wrap to ensure the correct body temperature is maintained.
- It moves latent heat for a longer period of time due to the longer exposure to the cold and wet conditions. This in turn creates movement of toxicity at a deeper level within the body.

NB As with the previous technique, do not use this technique where there is high blood pressure, pregnancy or a risk of haemorrhaging. Also avoid just after eating, as this may cause nausea.

To apply this technique you need:

- a normal household bath
- a body thermometer
- a small towel
- a cotton sheet (half the size of a single sheet or a single sheet folded in two)
- polythene sheets (to protect the bed)
- a hot water bottle (to help warm the body at the end of the technique)
- another person to help oversee the technique and to provide support if required.

Instructions:

1. Place the polythene sheets on your bed to protect it from the cold damp wrap.
2. Prepare the wrap by soaking a sheet in cold water, wringing it out and placing in the freezer for the duration of the hot tubbing stage.
3. Lie in a bath at a normal bath temperature.
4. Apply a cool wet towel to your head to ensure that it does not get too hot.
5. Add hot water to the bath at a gradual rate to begin raising the body temperature. Continue with this process until either the temperature has reached 102°F (38.9°C) or, prior to achieving that temperature, you feel that you are as hot as you are able to tolerate. (NB It is not safe to raise the body temperature to

more than 102°F unless you are in a supervised clinical environment.) Be sure to monitor your body temperature throughout by placing the thermometer in your mouth and to keep your head cool.

6. When you feel that you have had enough time in the hot water (every person's limits are different) or you have managed to maintain your body temperature at 102°F for 20 minutes, carefully get out of the bath.

7. Wrap yourself in the cold wrap (ideally from the neck to the feet, although usually from under the arms down to the thighs is more comfortable), then go to bed with a hot water bottle. Once in bed your body will start to mobilise latent heat in order to return its temperature to normal. Keep checking your temperature with the thermometer to ensure that it is increasing at a steady rate. Warm socks and hats can be used if required.

This technique has the same effect as a full-blown fever. It moves toxicity from a painful inflamed area out through the skin via the lymphatic system without challenging other vital organs and so can be useful in cases such as grumbling appendix or adhesions. It is interesting to note that the wrapping material can be discoloured by the end of the technique due to the toxic release through the skin.

Sitz Bath

This technique is very similar to the hot and cold showering but allows for more precise targeting of the pelvic region of the body. Like the hot and cold showering, it is aimed at creating movement within the circulatory system and thus within the lymphatic system.

Sitz baths bring both movement and energy to the reproductive system, bladder and bowel. In addition, the muscles relax when heated and contract when cooled, which can improve the muscle tone of these organs. Sitz baths are invaluable when you wish to stimulate movement within the pelvic organs. It is especially useful in muscular weakness, e.g. bladder weakness.

Do not apply this technique if there is any risk of haemorrhaging or during pregnancy.

To apply this technique you will need:

- **a normal household bath**
- **a small tub (such as a baby's bath).**

NB You can use two small tubs if there is no bath available.

Instructions:

1. **Fill the bath with hot water up to a level of about 5 inches (12.5 cm).**
2. **Fill the small tub with cold water up to a level of about 5 inches.**
3. **Sit in the hot water with your knees up for several minutes while continually splashing water over your lower torso.**

4. Change baths and sit in the cold water with your knees up for several minutes while continually splashing water over your lower torso.
5. Repeat this process three or four times and be sure to finish on cold.
6. Dry yourself with a towel, or with your hands if you want to create further movement.

Often after applying this technique the bowels or bladder need evacuating, due to the movement created.

This technique is very useful in cases of prolapsed organs, as the alternating hot and cold temperatures exercise the muscles by relaxing and contracting them. This exercise helps to tone the muscles and thereby keep the organs in the correct position. It also helps with hardening prostate, as the hot and cold temperatures stimulate movement within the blood and lymph and help to shift the stagnation that is contributing to the hardening.

Epsom Salts Bath

This technique focuses on the skin as a route of elimination. The skin is the largest organ of elimination and therefore can be an invaluable route through which to release toxicity, especially if the other organs of elimination are struggling. Epsom salts (magnesium sulphate) have the effect of drawing toxicity and acidity (especially uric acid) towards themselves. As a result, bathing in a high solution of Epsom salts draws toxicity from within the body out through the skin and into the solution.

It is interesting to note that Epsom salts were traditionally used to bring boils to a head and this clearly demonstrates this attraction between them and toxicity. The bath itself heats the body up, which opens up the cell membranes to release toxicity. It also thins the lymph, enabling it to help with the extra workload, and it encourages the blood to come to the surface of the skin. When Epsom salts and a hot bath are combined, they can produce a great deal of movement within the body to help remove toxicity.

Epsom salts have another very useful benefit because they are a sulphate. Within our bodies we need to convert the sulphur that we take in through our food into sulphate. In certain conditions, particularly in cases of autism, this conversion does not happen.

Magnesium in the sulphate form is very soothing, so simply adding Epsom salts to a bath can have a remarkably soothing effect on body and mind. It is especially helpful with children and young people with autism or behavioural problems.

This technique is beneficial for anyone who is undertaking a detoxification programme or has problems completing their daily elimination process. It is especially useful in soothing aching muscles or joints and so can be employed after heavy exertion or with conditions such as arthritis. Please note that it should not be applied if there is risk of haemorrhaging, high blood pressure or during pregnancy or menstruation.

Taking an Epsom salt bath once a week for three out of four weeks is a great way to ensure that the body keeps moving and releasing toxicity during the darker and more stagnant time of winter.

To apply this technique you will need:

- a normal household bath
- 2.2 lb (1 kg) of commercial Epsom salts (available from farm suppliers and garden centres).

Instructions:

1. Pour the Epsom salts into an empty bath.
2. Run the bathwater and agitate the salts to maximize the dissolving process. The bath should be warm to hot, depending on the intensity required. If running a hot bath, remember to wrap your head in a cool wet cloth.
3. Lie in the bath for up to 20 minutes (everyone's tolerance level is different, so be guided by how you feel). Do not use soap or add any other substance to the bathwater, as this can diminish the drawing out process.
4. Once you have reached your limit (or 20 minutes have passed), you can do any of the following:

- Add cold water to the bath to bring the temperature down and encourage the body to mobilise latent heat.
- Take a cold shower to encourage the body to mobilise latent heat.
- Quickly dry yourself and go to bed and continue sweating to encourage lymph movement and the release of toxins through the skin.

NB If using an Epsom salts bath with children, the bath temperature should only be warm and after the bath the child should be dried normally. This is a great technique to use with children before bedtime.

On completion of this technique, some people can feel a little weak and tired and so need to rest. After a good night's sleep, when the body has completed the induced elimination, people often feel very clear and refreshed.

Footbaths and Wraps

Footbaths have a less dramatic effect on the body than the full tubbing techniques but are able to concentrate their activity on a major area of elimination, namely the soles of the feet. This gentler effect can be very useful for people who need to take their healing process slowly at the beginning. Rather than subjecting the whole body to full tubbing, which creates a lot of change, you can start things moving gently by employing various types of footbath. This technique is also useful if you do not have a bath or cannot get into a bath due to a disability. It can easily be performed while sitting in a comfortable armchair.

Mustard Footbath

As with the tubbing techniques, a mustard footbath aims to create an artificial temperature within the body. This temperature thins the body fluids, creates movement and causes the body to sweat and detoxify through the skin. It is ideal if you want to start creating movement slowly within the body. As the effects are mild and the changes slow, it is an easy way to release toxins out of the body without overstressing it. This is an ideal technique to perform before bedtime.

To apply this technique you will need:

- a footbath (or a bowl the size of a washing-up bowl)
- English mustard powder
- a blanket.

Instructions:

1. Place a rounded dessertspoonful of English mustard powder into the footbath.
2. Add hot water to the bowl to a temperature that is comfortable.
3. Place your feet in the bowl to raise your temperature and begin the detoxification process.
4. If possible, place a blanket over your entire body, including the head, as this will help to induce an artificial fever for cleansing.
5. Remain in the footbath for 15–20 minutes (or less if you feel that you have had enough time).
6. Once you have completed your time in the footbath, dry your feet and go straight to bed to allow the elimination process to continue.

Epsom Salts Footbath

This technique is a milder and gentler version of the Epsom salts bath. It encourages the drawing of toxicity out through the skin and is also very soothing. Like the mustard bath, it is ideal before bedtime.

To apply this technique you will need:

- a footbath
- commercial Epsom salts
- a blanket.

Instructions:

1. Place 4 tablespoons of commercial Epsom salts into the footbath.
2. Add hot water to the bowl to a temperature that is comfortable.
3. Place your feet in the bowl to raise your temperature and begin the detoxification process.
4. If possible, place a blanket over your entire body, including the head, as this will help to induce an artificial fever for cleansing.
5. Remain in the footbath for 15–20 minutes (or less if you feel that you have had enough time).
6. Once you have completed your time in the footbath, dry your feet and go straight to bed to allow the elimination process to continue.

Cold Foot Wrap

This technique draws the blood supply down to the feet as the body seeks to warm them and restore the temperature balance within the body. As a result the rest of the body loses heat (especially the head).

This technique is very useful for two conditions. First, it is helpful in cases of fever if you wish to bring down the temperature of the head. Secondly, it is great if you suffer from an overactive mind before sleep. Many people do suffer from this, especially if their daily routine is stressful. This technique draws the blood away from the head and gives the brain the space to relax and induce a restful sleep.

To apply this technique you will need:

- one pair of cotton socks
- one pair of woollen socks.

Instructions:

1. Soak the cotton socks in cold water and wring them out until they are damp.
2. Place them in the freezer for 5–10 minutes.
3. Take them out of the freezer and put them on your feet.
4. Put the warm woollen socks over the top of them.
5. Go to bed and rest.

Castor Oil Packing

Castor oil has been known since ancient times for its healing properties. Known as the *Palma Christi*, or Palm of Christ, it was used extensively by Edgar Cayce in his work with patients.

It is difficult to find a complete explanation of why castor oil has such healing properties, but its results have been comprehensively documented. It is known to emit white light, which, like ordinary daylight, contains all the wavelengths of the visible spectrum at equal intensity. This white light penetrates the cell, giving it the energy to promote movement and thereby lessening the level of stagnation. In addition, it is known that the human cell produces its own measurable light in the form of bio-photons from within its DNA helix. It is my feeling that castor oil packing promotes the creation of this cellular light which the body can then use as energy for healing.

Castor oil packing is probably the ultimate technique for bringing energy to an area of the body that is struggling to shift stagnation. It is such a versatile technique that it benefits all situations, with the following exceptions: high blood pressure, during pregnancy or menstruation, or if there is a risk of haemorrhaging.

When applying castor oil packing there is a constant rule that should be applied in all situations: *wherever a problem area may be, you should always pack the liver first.* This ensures that this main route of elimination is open and ready to receive toxicity when it is released from the troubled area. Once the liver has been opened, you can apply a castor oil pack to the problem area to release the stagnation.

To apply this technique you will need:

- **a piece of unbleached brushed cotton or woollen material measuring 27 x 12 inches (67 x 30 cm)**
- **a bottle of castor oil (organic)**

- a roll of cling film or similar material
- a hot water bottle.

Instructions:

1. Fold the unbleached cotton into double or treble thickness.
2. Place it on a flat washable surface.
3. Pour on enough castor oil to cover it well but not so much that it starts to drip.
4. Place the oily cloth over the liver area.
5. Wrap cling film over the cloth and around your body to keep it in place.
6. Put on some old clothing in case of any leakages.
7. Relax and place a warm hot water bottle over the liver area and leave for one hour (in situations of extreme stagnation a longer duration may be required).
8. After you have packed the liver, you may repeat the process by packing any specific area of discomfort.

Castor oil packing is a powerful technique that will always create movement in the body. It should be applied with caution to anyone who suffers from high blood pressure. If in doubt, apply the pack initially for only 10 minutes in order to assess how you feel. Furthermore, because of the movement this technique creates, it may be useful to follow it with a further technique (e.g. an enema) in order to maintain the movement of toxicity through and out of the body.

On completion of this technique (and often during it), there is usually a feeling of deep relaxation. Pains and spasms are normally soothed and subside.

The frequency of castor oil packing will depend upon the situation, but I recommend that even in extreme cases this technique should not be implemented more than five days per week.

Areas that respond particularly well to packing are the liver, colon, lungs (on the front and the back) and reproductive areas, but any area of inflammation or toxicity will respond. Furthermore, the endocrine system, with its connection to light, also responds well to castor oil packing, so applying this technique to an area such as the thyroid can be most beneficial.

When castor oil packing is used after surgery it can prevent the formation of hard scar tissue and adhesions (the pack should be applied as soon as possible after the surgery). It likewise helps to relieve the discomfort of old scar tissue.

In cases such as bronchitis, castor oil packing to the lungs stimulates the movement of lymph and the draining of the congested lung tissue. Once again this should only be applied after first packing the liver.

Enemas

An enema is a very ancient technique in the world of healing and is an extremely powerful tool for bringing about swift change in both mind and body. The colon presents a very efficient route through which to bring therapeutic substances into the body because there is a direct connection between it and the liver. Whenever any substance, including all foods and liquids, enters the body, before it can be used it has to be marked as 'friendly' so that the immune system does not attack it, and it is within the liver that this labelling occurs, so the more quickly a substance arrives at the liver, the more quickly it can be used by the body. There is a large vein, called the portal vein, that connects the colon to the liver. Much of the absorption of nutrients from our food takes place in the small intestine and the colon or large intestine. The portal vein carries these nutrients to the liver, so anything that enters the colon via an enema will be similarly absorbed and transported via the portal vein directly to the liver. This makes enemas some of the most potentially potent and swift ways to bring about a change in the body biochemistry. The specific action of an enema will depend upon the therapeutic effect of the substance added to it.

Another function of the colon is eliminating waste products from the body. Waste matter is moved through the colon by a series of circular and spiralling muscle movements. Fibre is vitally important in the diet so that the muscles surrounding the colon wall have something to work with. A diet of highly refined over-processed foods that are low in fibre can lead to a weakening of this movement. This can mean that food does not pass efficiently through the system and can become stuck in the small pockets along the colon and impacted along the colon wall. This material then starts to ferment, making the colon very toxic. These toxins are then reabsorbed by the body, effectively overwhelming the liver with toxicity that it then has to try to store somewhere within the body. This is called 'auto-intoxication' and is the body poisoning itself with toxicity because it has no effective route of elimination open to it. Constipation is often the first sign of this problem. Similarly dehydration is registered in the colon and if someone is very dry, problems with constipation and the re-absorption of toxicity can arise.

Regular daily bowel movements are a sign of good health and enemas can greatly help to keep a sluggish bowel clean and the body hydrated while a purification and healing process is unfolding. Whenever there is a substantial release of toxins into the blood and lymph, an enema is the most effective way to carry those toxins out of the body. However, once health and balance are achieved, enemas should only be used as part of a health maintenance programme (e.g. once a week or once a month).

Many people are resistant to trying enemas, but they can be an extremely powerful way of speeding up the healing process and bringing both a physical and mental improvement.

NB Do not use enemas if there is a prolapsed organ in the pelvic area or if haemorrhoids are a problem.

How to Do an Enema

To apply this technique you will need:

- a gravity feed enema bag or bucket
- a 2-pint (1-litre) jug

- the fluid to be used for the enema (this will vary depending upon the type of enema, see below)
- a pillow
- something to protect the floor from liquid (towel or plastic sheet)
- lubrication (castor oil is very good)
- a hook upon which to hang the enema bag
- a clock for timing.

Instructions:

1. Prepare the enema fluid (as described in the specific enema types below).
2. Hang the enema bag/bucket on the hook so that the bottom of it is about 3 feet (1 metre) above the position you will lie in.
3. Check that the tap is closed then pour the enema fluid into the bag/bucket.
4. Release the air from the tube by allowing a small amount of liquid to run through.
5. Lubricate your anal area.
6. Prepare the floor area with protective material and then lie down on your back with your knees up or, if preferred, lie on your right side. The pillow can be used to support your head.
7. Insert the nozzle into your anus. (Some enema bags come with two different size nozzles. Use the smaller nozzle, as the larger one is designed for vaginal douching.)

8. Open the tap and allow the fluid to gently enter the rectal cavity. Massage your abdomen while the fluid is entering.
9. When all the fluid has entered, close the tap and remove the nozzle from your anus.
10. Hold the fluid for the specified time (as described in the specific enema types below). If you feel any discomfort, such as wind pains, massage your abdomen until it subsides.
11. On completion, move to the toilet to evacuate the enema.

Notes:

- A water enema may be advisable before any other enema to clear the bowel in preparation.
- If you have difficulty holding an enema, try reducing the fluid quantity and/or the holding time.
- Enemas often become easier if you are submerged in a bath of warm water, as the abdominal muscles are able to relax.
- It is not advisable to do enemas when hungry.
- It is not advisable to do stimulating enemas (e.g. coffee enemas) before bed.

Water Enema

If you have never experienced an enema before, a water enema is perhaps the best kind to start with. It introduces approximately 2 pints (1 litre) of water into the colon, which has a number of beneficial effects. It creates movement within the colon, encouraging it to release stored faeces. It also stimulates the reflex points within the colon. These points connect the colon to all other parts of the body. Stimulating these reflexes has the effect of releasing stagnation in areas of the body connected to these reflexes. Movement within the colon also stimulates movement and release of mucous from within the lymphatic system. Furthermore, some of the water held in the colon will be absorbed into the body, quickly helping to improve overall hydration.

Water enemas can be applied wherever the bowel is showing signs of constipation or where the lymphatic system is showing signs of stagnation (e.g. a cold or 'flu). They can also be useful when help is required to maintain the movement and release of toxicity during a cleansing programme or if you wish to improve the body hydration quickly (e.g. after a long-haul flight).

Often on completion of a water enema people feel light and refreshed. Sometimes light-headedness can occur. If so, rest is required. Occasionally, if the body is very dehydrated, the colon will retain all of the water so that no evacuation takes place.

Instructions:

1. **Prepare 2 pints (1 litre) of filtered water at body temperature. (It should be at body temperature because if it is too warm it will sedate the bowel and if it is too cool it will stimulate it.)**

2. Follow the instructions numbered 2–11 in 'How to Do an Enema' (*pages 185–187*).
3. Hold the water for 10–15 minutes.

Triple Water Enema

To apply three water enemas in sequence has a greatly increased effect. This technique is ideal at the onset of a cold, 'flu, sore throat or sinus congestion to bring extra stimulation to the lymphatic system. This extra stimulation will often ensure that the body does not need to create a full-blown fever in order to thin the lymph.

Often after completing this technique a person can feel rather drained and tired, so it is good to do it at the end of the day, as then you have the space to go to bed and rest.

If you suffer from a blocked head and sinuses at the onset of winter, it is sometimes useful to implement a triple water enema three times within 36 hours. This can often relieve congestion that might otherwise persist until the spring.

Instructions:

1. Prepare 2 pints (1 litre) of filtered water at body temperature.
2. Follow the instructions numbers 2–9 in 'How to Do an Enema' (*pages 185–187*).
3. Once all the water is in, massage the colon and then expel.

4. Repeat this process twice more (i.e. a total of three times).
5. The final water enema can be held for 10–15 minutes if desired.

Aloe Vera Enema

The water part of this enema does the same as described in the water enema technique. Aloe vera is moisturizing and soothing, so adding it to a water enema has an anti-inflammatory effect upon the mucosa of the colon. This makes it ideally suited to aiding any inflammatory conditions within the digestive system.

Often on completion of this technique a person feels calm and fresh, and it can have a very positive, softening effect upon the skin.

Instructions:

1. Prepare 2 pints (1 litre) of filtered water at body temperature.
2. Add between 1 and 10 tablespoons of aloe vera juice, depending upon the intensity required.
3. Follow the instructions numbered 2–11 in 'How to Do an Enema' (*pages 185–187*).
4. Hold for 15 minutes, massaging the colon throughout.

Coffee Enema

A coffee enema is perhaps the most powerful detox tool for the liver. It works in a unique way and is extremely useful once a purification programme is under way. The pharmacologically active part of the coffee is absorbed into the haemorrhoidal vein within the colon and is transported through the portal system directly to the liver. When the coffee arrives, it causes the liver to contract and squeeze its toxic bile out through the common bile duct into the duodenum and then out through the rest of the digestive tract. This contraction has a clearing effect upon the liver and leaves it in a much better state to continue with its detoxification role.

Because coffee enemas accelerate the liver's ability to detoxify, they reduce the risk of overload resulting in auto-intoxication. They can also be implemented in the case of an acute liver problem (e.g. migraines) to decongest the liver and bring about a quick solution.

On completion of this technique people can feel remarkably different in both mind and body. They often feel clear-headed and any aches and pains are reduced. They also feel less toxic, so have clearer vision and clearer thoughts and are in a better frame of mind. If there was any nausea before, this often disappears.

Coffee enemas can be useful if, for instance, you have done castor oil packing the night before and wish to contin-ue the movement of released toxicity. They have been used by the Gerson cancer therapy for decades due to their ability to help the body remove toxicity when tumours are breaking down.

You do need to be *very careful* with this technique, as it is one of the easiest to misunderstand. Coffee enemas do cause some loss of electrolytes (calcium, magnesium, sodium and potassium), which can cause stress in some cases. If overused or used in the wrong situation, they can bring about stress in the kidneys and adrenals due to this diuresis. As they have such profound effects, I always recommend that they are used only within a supervised programme. Instructions:

1. Place 1 rounded tablespoon of coarse ground organic coffee into a non-aluminium saucepan. (This measure can be reduced for a gentler effect.)
2. Pour on 0.5 pint (0.25 litre) of filtered water and bring to the boil.
3. Turn the heat down and simmer for 15 minutes, leaving uncovered.
4. Sieve into a 2-pint (1-litre) jug.
5. Make up to the required volume (1.5–2 pints/0.5–1 litre) with filtered water. Be sure to test that the fluid is at body temperature.
6. Follow the instructions numbered 2–11 in 'How to Do an Enema' (*pages 185–187*).
7. Hold for 15–20 minutes.

Choline Bitartrate Enema
It is not clear exactly how choline bitartrate (a B vitamin) acts when taken in the form of an enema, but in practice it seems to increase the efficiency of the liver. This technique is especially useful where any nausea is present. It can also be used as an alternative when a coffee enema should not be used (e.g. in a person who is very dehydrated, where

the loss of electrolytes could cause problems). Choline bitartrate is gentler on the kidneys and the adrenals than a coffee enema, so is useful when these areas need nurturing.

On completing this technique people often feel very clear. It can be useful in cases of recurring nephritis to effectively relieve intense nausea without stressing the kidneys and adrenals.

Instructions:

1. **Dissolve between 1 level teaspoon and 2 rounded teaspoons (depending on the intensity required) of choline bitartrate into a water enema.**
2. **Follow the instructions numbered 2–11 in 'How to Do an Enema' (*pages 185–187*).**
3. **Hold for 15–20 minutes.**

Chamomile Enema

Chamomile tea is a gentle sedative and when added to a water enema is absorbed via the haemorrhoidal vein (as with a coffee enema). It travels via the portal system to the liver and has a calming effect upon it and the rest of the body (i.e. the opposite effect to a coffee enema), so it is used to bring calmness to the liver, body and mind.

Often on completion of this technique people feel very calm, especially within the digestive system. It is very useful to have this enema in the evening before going to bed, as it aids restful sleep.

Instructions:

1. Put a rounded dessertspoon of organic chamomile flowerheads into a teapot and pour boiling water over them.
2. Leave to infuse for 20–30 minutes.
3. Sieve into a 2-pint (1-litre) jug.
4. Make up to 1.5–2 pints (0.5–1 litre) with filtered water. Be sure to test that the fluid is at body temperature.
5. Follow the instructions numbered 2–11 in 'How to Do an Enema' (*pages 185–187*).
6. Hold for 15–30 minutes.

Magnesium Enema

Magnesium is a muscle relaxant and has a generally soothing effect upon the body and mind. This makes a magnesium enema useful in situations where the muscles have gone into spasm (e.g. acute back pain), at the onset of a migraine if the early symptoms are neck and shoulder tension, and to relieve cramping at the onset of menstruation. It is also useful if there is muscle pain following rigorous exercise.

On completion of this technique people often experience a feeling of calm throughout their body. It is very common for any pains or spasms to disappear.

Instructions:

1. Dissolve 1–3 capsules of magnesium citrate (each capsule delivering 100mg of elemental magnesium) in a cup by pouring on hot water and stirring well. Total

dissolving is not possible, so there will be a powder residue on the top of the water.

2. Pour the magnesium solution into a 2-pint (1-litre) jug and make up to 1.5–2 pints (0.5–1 litre) with filtered water. Be sure to test that the fluid is at body temperature.

3. Follow the instructions numbered 2–11 in 'How to Do an Enema' (*pages 185–187*).

4. Hold for 15–30 minutes.

Flaxseed Tea Enema

This is an incredibly soothing enema that is useful for any kind of inflammatory bowel illness such as colitis or Crohn's disease. It is also wonderful for helping to bring hydration to the colon to relieve fear and anxiety and to help to stabilize blood sugar.

To make flaxseed tea:

● Place 2 tablespoons of flaxseeds (sometimes called 'linseeds') in a large non-aluminium pan.

● Add 2 pints (1 litre) of water and heat.

● Bring to the boil, immediately take off the heat and cover.

● Let the mixture stand for 12 hours or overnight.

● Return the pan to the heat and gently simmer with the lid off for 1 hour.

● Immediately sieve the tea and discard the seeds.

● The thick liquid can be stored in the fridge once cooled if it is not being used immediately.

Instructions:

1. Mix the flaxseed tea with warm water, bringing the mixture to body temperature and to a consistency that makes it easy to pass through an enema tube.
2. Follow the instructions numbered 2–11 in 'How to Do an Enema' (*pages 185–187*).
3. Hold for 15–20 minutes.

Flaxseed Oil Enema
Flaxseed oil enemas promote a great deal of photon and electron activity within the body. This technique can be useful at the start of a healing programme to bring more light and electrons into the body. Dr Johanna Budwig would give this enema as her first prescription. It can be used in situations where people are unable to take oil orally due to digestive difficulties or where they are unable to utilize oils (e.g. in people with ME). It is also useful at times of high energy (e.g. at equinoxes) to maximize their effects.

On completion of this technique people often feel an incredible sense of calmness and connectedness. It is very powerful and is usually only performed occasionally, e.g. once a month or once a year.

Instructions:

1. Warm a bottle (9–17 fl.oz/250–500ml) of organic flaxseed oil to body temperature by placing it into a jug of warm water.

2. Follow the instructions numbered 2–11 in 'How to Do an Enema' (*pages 185–187*).
3. Hold for 60 minutes.
4. Follow the flaxseed oil enema with a water enema to clear the colon of oil.
5. Pour hot soapy water through the enema bag afterwards to clean out any oil residue.

Flaxseed Oil Implant (mini enema)

A flaxseed oil implant is similar to the previous technique but acts over a longer period of time. Like the flaxseed oil enema, it can be useful where people cannot take oils orally due to digestive difficulties or cannot break down oils effectively, or at times of natural high energy (e.g. at equinoxes).

On completion of this technique and after a good night's sleep people often feel very calm, as if the whole nervous system has benefited.

To apply this technique you will need:

- an implant pipette
- 0.5–2 fl.oz (15–60ml) of organic flaxseed oil.

Instructions:

1. Warm the required amount of flaxseed oil to body temperature by placing the bottle of oil into a jug of warm water.
2. When the oil is warm, draw it up into the pipette.
3. Lubricate your anal area.

4. Insert the nozzle and squeeze the bulb of the pipette so that it pushes the oil into the rectal area. Be sure to keep the bulb compressed constantly until all of the oil has entered and the nozzle has been removed.
5. Ideally, hold overnight.

Clysmatics

Clysmatics were developed by one of Sweden's original naturopaths, Birger Ledin, and have been used safely in homes, clinics and hospitals throughout Sweden for over 70 years. The system is medically approved in Sweden and is easily used. It fits into the toilet so that the whole technique is performed while sitting on the toilet. It does not weaken the natural defecation reflexes and because the liquid is fed into you under only the pressure of gravity, it is much gentler than a colonic (see the next technique). The equipment is easily packed away and stored, so this technique can be utilized discreetly.

Clysmatics push a gently pressured flow of water into the colon, which is allowed to build up until a strong desire to empty the colon is created. Once emptied, the colon refills with water until another release is required. This process is repeated several times. The unique design of the clysmatic allows the inflow nozzle to remain in the anus while the bowel evacuation is taking place. This design feature protects the clean water that is waiting to enter the colon from the evacuation by use of a one-way valve. This allows the technique to be completed without the need for re-insertion.

This constant flushing of water in and out of the colon removes mucous and faeces. The main purpose of the technique, however, is to stimulate all the reflexes within the colon. This stimulation is similar to an internal massage and has the potential to create movement and release in all parts of the body.

This technique can be very useful where consistent constipation is a problem, as it will help to clear the bowel and tone the muscles, helping to re-educate the bowel. It is also useful during a cleansing programme to help stimulate deep tissue release and in stagnant lymphatic situations (e.g. a cold, 'flu or a sore throat).

On completion of this technique people can feel light-headed, in which case rest is recommended.

To apply this technique you will need:

- 1 clysmatic
- 9–14 pints (5–8 litres) of filtered water.

Instructions:

1. Set the clysmatic up as described in the manufacturer's instructions.
2. Fill the container with 9–14 pints (5–8 litres) of water at body temperature.
3. Lubricate the anal region.
4. Sit on the nozzle.
5. Open the tap to allow water to flow through.
6. While water is entering, contract the anal sphincter, allowing the water to fill up the colon.

7. When the pressure in the colon begins to become uncomfortable, release the anal sphincter to release the bowel contents.
8. Repeat this process until the reservoir of water is emptied.

You can also add any of the substances that you can add to enemas, apart from oil, to enhance the therapeutic effects of the water.

Colonics

A colonic passes 26 pints (15 litres) of water through the colon. The speculum used enables water to flow in and waste to leave simultaneously. The water is built up to fill the entire colon by pinching the waste pipe. When the water reaches the ileocoecal valve at the far end of the colon, the colon creates an energetic flush, pushing the contents of the colon out through the waste pipe.

The first 9 pints (5 litres) of water are administered with the client lying on their left side so that the cleansing mainly takes place in the descending colon. The second and third 9 pints (5 litres) are usually administered with the client lying on their back (with their knees up), so that the water can reach the far side of the colon. This position also enables the abdomen to be massaged to facilitate a better colon cleanse.

The constant flushing of water in and out of the colon removes mucous and faeces. Like the clysmatic, however, the main purpose of this technique is to stimulate all the reflexes within the colon to create movement and release in all parts of the body.

This technique can be very useful where consistent constipation is a problem, as it will clear the bowel and tone the muscles, helping to re-educate the bowel. It can be helpful during a cleansing programme to help deep tissue release, in stagnant lymphatic situations and before and after a fast. Some people use this technique at the spring equinox to give the body a kick-start in taking full advantage of the cleansing properties of spring.

On completion of this technique some people can feel tired and light-headed and some can feel quite toxic for the following few days. To apply this technique you will need to make an appointment with a colonic therapist.

Urine Therapy

What I have found in my travels to different parts of the world when I have talked with the local people is that all of the old cultures practised urine therapy. Using urine as a healing tool dates back thousands of years. It has many different applications, from treating wounds and burns to changing the charge around the cell membrane. It is used both externally and internally, but it is the external use of urine that I have found particularly useful in my work.

Urine is basically an overflow of the lymphatic system and is completely sterile when passed unless there is a specific urinary or kidney infection. The use of urine as a therapy is called *isopathy*, meaning 'identical treating identical', as opposed to *homoeopathy*, which is 'like treating like'. Your urine holds within it all the information of who you really are, along with a rich mixture of vitamins and minerals. It is very useful for both drawing out toxicity and cleansing.

When using urine externally, collect your first passing of the day. The old Indian urine therapists used to say of this morning collection, 'Reject the head and tail of the serpent.' This means that you collect the urine midstream. Pour it into a glass bottle and allow the air to get to it by lightly placing a cotton wool bung in the top of the bottle. Don't put it in the fridge, but store it in a cool dark place for a minimum of three days. The urine is now ideal to use externally because it has undergone a chemical change. As it is exposed to the air, it becomes more alkaline and this gives it the property of drawing inflammation out of the body. It does this by drawing sodium out of the cells and out through the skin. This makes urine rubbing the quickest way to change the charge around the cell membrane and therefore the overall body charge. Externally, urine is used that is 3–10 days old. This has both a cleansing and an anti-inflammatory effect.

Full-Body Urine Rubbing

Instructions:

1. Warm up a bottle of 3–10-day-old urine by placing the bottle in a jug of warm water. Pour the warmed urine into a bowl (classically this was a copper container).
2. Sit in your bath or shower and begin by wetting your bare hands with urine and rubbing the urine into your face and neck until they are dry (i.e. until the urine has absorbed and the skin is dry).
3. Next rub urine into both feet, top and bottom, again until the skin is dry.

4. Work your way up your body, reaching all the parts you can, and always rubbing the urine in until the skin is dry. Some areas will absorb it more quickly than others. It works on the high elimination areas well, but you can be random in your application.
5. When you have rubbed urine into your entire body (front and back), once again rub your face and neck until the skin is dry.
6. Have a shower or bath and wash with a natural soap.

Obviously this process can take some time. Indeed, in an ideal situation you would rub for an hour. However, if you are short of time, try just rubbing the face, neck, soles of the feet and palms, as these are the main outlet areas of the skin.

It is very nice as part of a general maintenance programme to do a skin brush followed by a 20-minute full-body urine rub and then finish off with some hot and cold showering. This makes an excellent way to kick-start your day, especially if you have a lot to do.

Full-body urine rubbing can be done weekly or daily, depending on the intensity of the movement required. It is particularly useful for people who are unable to draw toxicity out of the body via enemas.

Urine Packing

Urine packing can have an amazing effect upon the body and packing the kidneys is especially powerful. I have known people with nephritis who, within an hour of applying a urine pack to their kidneys, have had a dramatic reduction in their symptoms. In this situation, even packing with fresh urine (if no old urine is available) can be most helpful.

In our study of the five elements we learned that the kidneys were the seat of fear, so packing the kidneys with urine can be very helpful when people are in a state of high anxiety or fear. I have also noticed this to be particularly useful in cases of ulcerative colitis, where I can often hear the fear and anxiety in the voice of the person. In these situations I often recommend that the person initially applies a urine pack to their kidneys every evening for a minimum of an hour and continues with this practice until their level of fear and anxiety subsides.

To apply this technique you will need:

- **a small piece of unbleached brushed cotton or similar cloth about the size of a tea towel**
- **a bottle of your own urine that is 3–10 days old**
- **a roll of cling film or similar material.**

Instructions:

1. Warm the urine up by placing the bottle in a jug of warm water.
2. Pour the urine onto the cloth, making sure the whole area is wet.
3. Wring out any excess urine and apply the pack to the kidney area (the mid to lower back).
4. Cover the pack in cling film to prevent leakage.

5. **Lie down and relax for an hour.**
6. **Remove the pack and wash or shower.**

NB There is *no* need to apply extra heat (e.g. a hot water bottle) to a urine pack.

Urine packs can be applied to all sorts of other areas of the body with great effect. In situations where women have had the lymph nodes under their arms removed, urine packing to the underarms helps to open up a route of elimination and ease lymph blockages in this area. Another area that responds very powerfully to urine packing is the thyroid. If someone has an underactive thyroid, full body rubbing combined with packing to the thyroid can be very helpful. I find that a half-hour castor oil pack followed by a half-hour urine pack to the thyroid can bring a lot of healing energy to this area. The lungs, especially when congested, also respond very favourably to urine packing, as does any area that is swollen or inflamed.

Fresh urine can be used almost anywhere on the body. It can be used in a footbath to help to draw toxicity out through the soles of the feet, for example. It is also remarkable for curing most types of earache. If a child has an earache, try placing a couple of drops of its own or its mother's fresh urine in the ears. It is wonderful for the eyes (try bathing your eyes morning and evening with fresh urine or placing a couple of drops in each eye). This is one of the best ways I have found to quickly and effectively treat conjunctivitis. When used in a nasal douche (sometimes called a neti), urine greatly helps to clear the sinuses. Fresh urine placed in the hair and left for an hour before washing (cover the head in a towel) has a great softening effect and improves the quality of the hair and scalp. Indeed, one of the chief components of urine, urea, is used in a great many commercial hair and skin products. This urea is invariably collected from the urine of animals. Surely it is much preferable to use your own? It is quite common after someone has begun the practice of urine rubbing to find that people comment on how healthy and vital their skin looks.

Internal Urine Therapy

Drinking your own urine can have a remarkable effect on your body and mind and has been practised for thousands of years. Indeed, it is a much more common practice even today than you might at first imagine. Once again it is the morning passing, midstream, that is traditionally used.

If you want to start gently I recommend just rinsing your mouth out with some fresh morning urine, which is also one of the most effective treatments I know for gingivitis and bleeding gums. Then you might like to try gargling with morning urine.

When it comes to actually drinking urine, I recommend that at first you start with a few sips of fresh urine taken midstream in the late afternoon, as this will be milder than the morning passing. You can then increase the amount of this urine that you drink and once you feel comfortable, switch to drinking the first passing of the morning.

When drinking your own urine you need to be very aware of what I call the 'push and pull'. If you are drinking urine, which is your true vibration, it will create a process of detoxification as your body begins to release substances that do not hold your vibration. If you are doing this cleansing work from within, it is also important to do urine rubs so that you pull the toxicity out from the body through the skin. This is what I mean when I talk about matching the push and pull. This also makes the use of urine one of the most powerful of all the techniques. Furthermore, it is completely free and readily available anywhere because you always have urine with you.

NB Taking urine internally is not recommended for those who eat much meat or take regular medication.

All of the above techniques can be very powerful and very healing when employed at the correct time, but they do need to be used wisely. Your feelings are your best guide. Only do a technique when it feels right to do so. Techniques should not be applied randomly in the hope of bringing about change. They should be applied with a clear understanding of which specific areas need support or targeting.

Techniques are really all about helping you to connect at a deeper level with who you really are. When you give the body extra tools like these to aid its cleansing and healing process, it will reward you with a deeper connection with yourself. As you use them, your intuition will become stronger, so that you will feel when it is the right time to practise a technique and will intuitively know which technique to perform, for how long and with the exact level of intensity to suit you at that particular moment in time. Techniques can greatly ease the extra pressure placed upon the body during the healing process and are all potentially hugely consciousness altering.

CHAPTER 10

FINAL THOUGHTS

We live in an amazing universe made up of vibrating energy that is forever changing and expanding. Nothing remains the same; the only constant is change. Anything within the universe that tries to resist this change will create stress and friction. On a human level we know that when there are stress and friction between two individuals, there are likely to be conflict and dis-ease. Likewise, when there are stress and friction between us and the universal energies, internal conflict and dis-ease are inevitable.

We were designed to stand on the leading edge of reality, to dare to dream new and wonderful dreams and to hold within us the power to make those dreams reality. Our thoughts and dreams are vibrations that we continually send out into the universe and these vibrations will either resonate or be out of phase with the unfolding energies of the universe. Because the universe is forever expanding, any thought or dream that is expansive will naturally resonate in harmony with all that is. Similarly, any thought that is contractive will be out of phase and cause friction and stress. Simply put, if you want to be happy, healthy and free, all you need to do is think and dream only about things that make you feel good.

Our emotions are the language we use to communicate with the universe and the universe always mirrors back to us whatever we express. If we think predominantly negative and fearful thoughts, the reality that is mirrored back to us is one of stress and fear. If we think predominantly positive, happy thoughts, our reality becomes one of peace, joy and beauty. What you experience in the world is always a reflection of how you feel. So if you are suffering in any way from dis-ease, whether it is a general dissatisfaction with life or a life-threatening illness, the guide on your path back to balance is your emotions. If you seek thoughts, feelings and experiences that consistently make you feel better, you will find a quality of life beyond your dreams.

The key lies in consistency. There are many things in life that give the illusion of making us feel better, such as a bar of chocolate or a drug, but if you really want to feel better you must look within. If you can understand how layers of toxicity have, over time, taken you further away from who you really are, you will have understood the fundamental root of all dis-ease. What's more, with the information I have shared with you in this book, you have everything you need to gently release that toxicity and rediscover just what an amazing being you are.

The human body never ceases to thrill me with its wonderful integrity and design. It is a vehicle that was perfectly designed to transport us in this physical reality on a magical adventure of pure expansion. It was built to self-repair and to always be able to return, given the right circumstances, to a place of balance and harmony.

The body has many windows into its innermost workings for those able to see through them. The eyes are often referred to as 'the windows to the soul', but to an iridologist they are also a window into the innermost workings of every part of the body. A traditional Chinese acupuncturist will use windows provided through the pulse, tongue and face to see where there is an interruption in the free flow of energy around the body. All traditional medicine men and women throughout the world know about these windows and indeed so does every human being on this planet, even if they are not aware of it. If you go into partnership with your body and begin to work with it rather than against it, you will be rewarded with access to these windows. Your body wants to show you how to bring it back into balance and harmony and your intuition and feelings are the key. You do not need to become an expert in medicine, ancient or modern, to become whole. You only need to become an expert in who you really are.

We are vibrational beings and we need to vibrate in harmony with our universe if we are to fulfil our true potential. It is time for us to come to understand what it means to be in resonance so that we can beat and pulse together instead of living in this world that we have created where everything is in opposition. The changes that are currently taking place have created the possibility of bringing this potential into reality. The pulse of the Earth is speeding up. The Schumann resonance is now high compared to what it was in the past. The level of photon vibration is increasing all the time, so that it becomes much easier to see the truth once your eyes are open. The challenge for us is to match our microcosm to the macrocosm. We too need to raise our vibration, our consciousness, and allow the light of the universe to illuminate the beauty of who we really are. We need to stop resisting and surrender to our cellular awakening. It is our destiny. These changes are here and we have to face them whether we like it or not. We have to realize that we have the power to bring about massive change for the good of all. There is no more sitting on the fence. We each have to take responsibility and choose how we want the world to be. Do you want to live in a continuation of what has been or would you like to live in a beautiful world of peace, harmony and forever expanding happiness? Are you going to continue to allow fear and confusion to be your dominant feelings or would you rather have love, compassion and understanding as your reality?

Every one of us knows on some level that we were born to be happy, but that happiness can only be realized when we dance in harmony with creation. The incredible quickening of these vibrations in our universe is here to help us, not to challenge us. The challenge only comes when we refuse to accept our destiny to fulfil our true potential.

Peace is the experience of balance and harmony and comes to us only when we all vibrate together. We know that when we are in a peaceful, loving state, it is absolutely amazing. There is a harmony of vibration, the resonances completely matching. This is the energy created between mother and baby after the moment of birth. The mother looks lovingly at her own creation and sees pure love mirrored back to her. One of the most thrilling experiences we can have is to be witness to the birth of new life, for it reminds us of the wonder and beauty of who we really are. We were each born to be the deliberate creators of our own reality and to make that reality one of fun, laughter, joy and beauty. We are expansive beings and co-creators of an expanding universe. How you feel is your simple but powerful guide to what you are calling into your reality. When we are vibrating in harmony with the universe, we feel at one and this allows for expansion. When we are pushing against the universe, life becomes difficult and challenging. The time has come to stop struggling and striving for happiness and to just allow ourselves to flow easily into it.

All of the problems in the world have arisen out of our separation from one another. We are each living in such different realities that it is becoming almost impossible to communicate with those outside our own vibration. All conflict in this world has arisen out of an inability to effectively communicate with one another. From broken relationships to world wars, all disputes have arisen from a lack of resonance with one another.

This is reflected in ourselves when we manifest dis-ease. When a part of the body malfunctions, that part is not in resonance with the rest of the body. If, for example, there is dis-ease within the lungs, the ability to hold and express grief and the aspiration for purity will not be moving smoothly. We need to be able to bring that part of the body back into resonance.

We cannot raise our consciousness if there is friction between any part of our being or between us and the space-time we occupy. When the body is not well, it needs lovingly nurturing back to harmony. If we want to live in peace and harmony with one another, if we want to lead lives filled with meaning and adventure, if we want to truly fulfil our monumental potential as co-creators of our reality, we must each learn to come back into resonance with the universal laws.

Often I find that when a situation arises for which I cannot immediately find a solution, turning everything on its head presents a new perspective which often brings the solution into focus. In doing this we really start to look at things differently. Many people think that matter influences consciousness, for instance, but think for a moment of consciousness as the creator of matter. When we look at the world from this perspective we begin to understand how we create our own reality and just how much influence we can have on our lives.

I love unusual perspectives because they make you think in new and expansive ways. One such perspective is that the sun doesn't actually produce heat and light, but in fact its function is to reflect the consciousness emanating from the Earth. Such a perspective helps us to hold and own the fact that we are the creators and participants in an amazing unfolding story. Just ponder for a moment how this world would be if we turned our perspective on its head. What if, rather than fighting against bacteria and viruses, we went into partnership with them? What if we no longer viewed them as enemies but as allies within our body to aid us in our perpetual seeking of balance, harmony and resonance? What a change that would bring to our understanding of disease.

We are each living in a human body, but now perhaps it is time for us to realize our position within the greater universe. There are many courses you can do and books you can read relating to the physical world, such as those about nutrition, agriculture and animal husbandry, and equally there is a huge range of subjects relating to the spiritual path. But what is more interesting is the fact that we live between these two energies, the physical and the spiritual. We are at the very core of this whole process called 'life'. Once we become aware of this, we can begin to see things much more clearly and to take responsibility for our own lives. This personal responsibility aspect is what we have been talking about repeatedly throughout this book. It is both our sole responsibility and our soul responsibility to prepare our vehicle so that it communicates and radiates the universal energies. We need to understand how to work with the earthly *and* heavenly energies and encompass them in the meeting place that is our body.

The upper energies of heaven and the lower earthly energies come together in food. This has been largely forgotten in our modern society. The growing of food has become so distanced from where we actually live and in many cases has become more and more distanced from any human contact. Our ancestors understood the power of making a connection with the land and the food they grew upon that land. If we reclaimed this knowledge, our experience of food would be completely different. When *you* plant a seed with *your* own hand, *your* DNA and therefore *your* vibration is left on that seed. As you tend the growing plant, your vibration is continually interacting with the vibration of that plant and the land in which it is growing. When you harvest and eat that plant, it becomes your own unique medicine infused with the vibrations of heaven, Earth and you. As your body digests this food, there is no resistance, no stress.

Nature is a great balancer and will provide in any given area all of the plants needed to bring nourishment and healing to the people living in that area. This healing and nourishing power is greatly enhanced when the people interact with the plants and the land. This is what Rudolf Steiner meant when he suggested that if we want to heal ourselves, we must first heal the Earth. There is a need for us to be involved in all of the processes of our nutrition.

When you make a connection with heaven and Earth, when you respect the land and dance with the universal energies, you also make a deeper connection to who you really are. You develop an inner knowing that the solution to every problem lies within you.

Rudolf Steiner told a wonderful story that demonstrates this beautifully. It involves someone living in Austria who grew their own food, following biodynamic principles. Biodynamic farming is founded on the understanding that we stand between heaven and Earth. Seeds are planted, tended and harvested in harmony with the moon and other universal energies. This person had no formal medical knowledge or training in the medicinal use of plants. However, when one day they developed a stomach problem, they knew intuitively which of their plants they needed to eat to bring about a cure. In this case it was a particular white cabbage. There was an inner knowing that the cabbage held the vibration that would relieve the stomach problem. They had planted it, so their vibration was planted with it. When they ate it, the vibration of the cabbage within their body was able to shift the block of the dis-ease and bring the body immediately back a place of harmony. To some this might seem magical, but it is a magic that we each hold within us. When we grow food that is in resonance with us individually, there is no resistance.

Cellular awakening is a wonderful journey of self-illumination. By giving our cells the right nourishment, we awaken our potential to connect with universal wisdom. And although for each one of us the story unfolds differently, the journey of discovery takes all of us to a place of pure bliss. It is a receiving and passing of wisdom from one being to another and so on in the same way that light travels from cell to cell.

You have found a new way of looking at your amazing body and how it really works. You have listened to your own story and interpreted it. You have understood how to bring yourself back to harmony. You know how to connect and awaken your cells and you have the tools to make it reality. So where do you want to go next?

APPENDIX I

THREE MINI CASE HISTORIES

Once we begin to apply the principles of cellular awakening to a case history, the connections in someone's story begin to reveal themselves. We begin to see how the levels of dehydration and stress have gradually gone deeper and to take note of the many times the body has tried to redress the imbalance. We observe Hering's Law in action and how the body has danced with the natural rhythms. As this process unfolds, we begin to perceive the amazing integrity of the body and to understand how nature provides us with all the energies we need to heal. To give you a taste of how a story can connect, there follow three different case histories with interpretations. They show three different ways in which the tubercular taint can show itself. These are not full case histories but the highlighted events in each person's life that were the most powerful connecting points in their story.

Mini Case Number I

- Breech presentation at birth.
- No breastfeeding.
- All vaccines given.
- Ear infections treated with antibiotics.
- BCG vaccination coinciding with the onset of puberty.
- Glandular fever.
- After glandular fever always very achy and arthritic. Sleep becomes a problem – goes to bed late and gets up late. Symptoms of ME.

Interpretation

When a baby presents incorrectly it is due to the fact that the charge in the mother's uterus is not correct, so the placenta has embedded in the wrong place. We know from our understanding of the day/night exchange that a change in charge can occur only if there is dehydration present within the mother. When dehydration is present, the cell will protect itself by building a cholesterol layer, which will in turn impede the exchange of electrolytes within that cell. There will be a build-up of the wrong electrolytes within the cell and the day/night exchange will not fully take place.

In a dehydrated mother this change in charge creates a change in the polarity of the uterus. When the polarity of the uterus is correct, the placenta attaches itself to the top of the uterus so that the umbilical cord hangs down, allowing the developing child to dance freely. When the polarity is not strong enough, the placenta embeds at the side of the uterus and it is this situation that leads to the wrong presentation at birth. In more extreme cases the placenta can embed across the birth canal or even outside the womb in a Fallopian tube, leading to an ectopic pregnancy. When a mother is dehydrated, some of this dehydration will also be passed on to her baby.

No breastfeeding means that the copper–zinc ratio would not have been corrected, which can cause problems with dependency. Furthermore, breastmilk helps the baby to develop the correct bowel flora, which does not occur when an alien product such as formula milk is introduced from birth.

Vaccinations bring vibrational stress into the baby, which will increase dehydration further. Often when this occurs, it is easy within a full case history to see an imbalance in the five elements beginning to show, especially the Metal element. The baby might show the first signs of constipation, skin problems such as eczema or even a change in behaviour (e.g. not sleeping so well or having less energy). The depth of the manifestation (whether it is showing in skin, colon, lungs or mind) is a clear indicator of the depth of dehydration. When dehydration increases, you can also often notice an increase in acute illnesses as the body attempts to clear toxicity that has accumulated as a result of the day/night exchange not fully taking place. In this case history this shows itself as ear infections. In the five elements system there is a connection between the ears and the kidneys and both are governed by the Water element, so we can see an increase in the level of dryness in this person. Antibiotics would have not only suppressed the illness and taken it deeper into the body, but would also have affected body temperature, so we can see that the conditions within the test tube are deteriorating.

By the time this person reaches puberty, their body is clearly already struggling to maintain balance. Giving the BCG vaccine, which is the tubercular vaccine, at the onset of puberty superimposes an energy picture of disease onto this person. If they are carrying the tubercular taint within their predisposition, this vaccine can bring that taint from the past (the ancestry) into the present. It is very common for this to manifest as glandular fever, as it does in this case. Glandular fever only arises in a person who is really struggling to clear away toxicity. It is also very common for people to 'never be well since' having glandular fever. This is a sign that the lymphatic system and liver are both becoming congested, and this always has a direct effect upon energy levels. This is followed by symptoms of arthritis and achiness, which are both signs of increased toxicity and with it a change in pH. The person is becoming more acidic.

After this it is clear that the higher aspects of this person have become affected, as shown by sleep problems ('I can't sleep' is higher than 'My joints hurt'). Their natural body clock no longer dances with the sun and the moon and they find themselves going to bed late and getting up late. This is a clear sign of a deeper level of interruption to the day/night cycle and hence a deeper level of dehydration. By this time the person would have lost the ability to create acute responses to release toxicity, so it is not surprising that they have all the symptoms of ME.

Mini Case Number 2

- Very high birth weight.
- Breastfed for three months.
- Usual vaccinations given.
- Ear infection – treated with antibiotics.
- Onset of menstruation – very irregular.
- One year after menarche the BCG vaccination given.
- Within six months of BCG, eating distress.
- In her twenties, polycystic ovaries.

Interpretation
In this case we have a baby with a very high birth weight. This is an indication of a predisposition to diabetes, which is both an extreme blood sugar issue and an endocrine imbalance. Blood sugar imbalances are linked to the body's inability to hold calcium in the correct place, which in turn is linked to dehydration, so it is likely that this person was born with a pre-existing level of dehydration passed down the family lines. This inherited dehydration predisposes her to blood sugar imbalances and hence ultimately to diabetes. However, she would need to create deeper levels of

dehydration for diabetes to actually manifest. From our study of Hering's Law we know that disease rises up the body from the bottom to the top. In this case we can see that the endocrine imbalance has only reached the reproductive area and has not yet risen to the level of the pancreas. Remember that endocrine imbalance is linked to a lack or imbalance of essential fatty acids, so it is also likely that this person was born with an inherited lack or imbalance of these vital nutrients. She was breastfed for the first three months, but one has to remember that the quality of the breastmilk is equal only to the quality of the mother's diet at that time. Then we can see that the implementation of the usual vaccination programme would have brought a lot of stress to the body and therefore created deeper levels of dehydration. This means that the person would have become dryer and more disconnected from all of the natural rhythms that the body normally dances with. The ear infections would have been the body's attempt to throw off toxicity, but with the suppressive treatment of antibiotics this process would not have taken place.

As this person reaches puberty, we see that menstruation is irregular, showing clearly how disconnected she has become from the rhythm of the moon. From our work on the five elements we can see that this also implicates the liver and gall bladder, because things in the body are not going to plan. Furthermore we can surmise that there will be a lack of the essential ingredients in the nutrition to look after the endocrine system, the hydration and the pH.

At this stage, the irregular menstruation is a sign that

things are not right, but the symptoms have not yet reached a serious and disruptive stage. However, once the BCG vaccination is given, we can quickly see a deterioration, as manifested by the eating distress. We can see that prior to this she was already struggling to maintain health. The stress of this vaccine would have pushed her to a point where she had eating distress. This often manifests as periods of bingeing on foods containing high levels of refined carbohydrates (wheat and sugar especially), salt and denatured fats. She would therefore have experienced dramatic crashes in blood sugar levels and extreme and irresistible food cravings as her predisposition to blood sugar imbalance came more and more to the fore.

Finally, in her twenties, she receives a diagnosis of polycystic ovaries. If this were further suppressed, it is almost inevitable that diabetes would appear later on in life.

Fortunately, once this person was reconnected to who she really was, she understood how to walk a path back to health and to begin to write a new story of ever-improving health.

Mini Case Number 3

- Normal birth.
- Syntometrin given to the mother at birth (this is a drug given during the third stage of labour to speed up the delivery of the placenta, which often leads to jaundice in the baby).
- Breastfed for a short time.

- All vaccinations given.
- Throat infections, treated with antibiotics.
- BCG vaccination coincides with the beginning of puberty.
- IBS during teens.
- Bad acne treated three times each with a six-month course of oxytetracycline (an antibiotic).
- Very low energy at the end of puberty.
- Huge weight issues.

Interpretation

In this third case we have a situation where although the birth is normal, the drug Syntometrin is given in order to speed up placental deliveries. This drug is administered while the baby is still connected to the mother via the umbilical cord. It interferes with the natural plan of the mother's birth process and therefore affects the liver ('the planner') of both mother and child. This manifests in the baby as jaundice, which is a liver disorder and a sure sign of stress and dehydration. Then this child is only breast-fed for a short time and the introduction of formula milk, which is an unnatural product, at such a young age will have added further stress. Vaccines will have increased the stress, so it is little surprise that throat infections manifest as a means of the body trying to clear toxicity. When these are treated with antibiotics, there is another increase in stress, dehydration and the suppression of potential. Throat infections show that there is a stagnation of the lymph which the body is trying to clear with an acute illness. When this illness is suppressed, the stress, dehydration and toxicity inevitably go deeper into the body.

Then in this story we move into puberty, which we know is a challenging time, and once again the tubercular BCG vaccine is given. This will certainly have a huge impact on an already stressed body and we see both the colon and skin showing problems. In the five elements these two organs are part of the Metal element and are strongly implicated in tubercular pictures. The irritable bowel syndrome shows that the colon is not able to clear in a normal manner due to chronic dehydration. Then the body, in its perfect integrity, tries to push toxicity out through the skin (acne). The acne is suppressed with long-term use of antibiotics on three occasions, with no one actually looking at the connections between the colon, skin, liver and lymph unfolding in this person's story. Long-term use of antibiotics creates a lot of depletion because antibiotics disrupt the natural bowel flora and therefore disrupt both digestion and absorption. By the end of puberty this person has become so deficient and had such an unbalanced digestive system that low energy and weight issues manifest.

So often in a situation such as this, no one makes a connection between all these aspects and so the story is not understood and the solution impossible to locate. But it never ceases to amaze me how quickly people can turn their own story around and start to heal once they understand how and why they have arrived at the place of dis-ease.

APPENDIX II

IODINE

Historically we have moved from being shoreline and estuary dwellers and we need to consider what we might have lost nutritionally as a consequence of this. We are obviously eating far less fish and fewer sea vegetables and all of the other foods that naturally exist in the shoreline environment. It has been seen that people who live and eat by the sea, particularly people living on islands, have a very high intake of iodine each day within their diet. They also show remarkably good health, with very low rates of cancer, heart disease and the many other health problems that seem to trouble modern society. In recent times a lot of research and many surveys have been done which have come to the conclusion that we each need to take in at least 12.5 mg of iodine a day either in our diets or as supplementation. Clinicians in the past have used 37.5 mg a day and in some cases dramatically higher doses.

Iodine has long been linked to thyroid function, but in reality it is required by every single cell within our bodies. Iodine levels are found to be naturally high in certain areas of the body, such as the thyroid, the ovaries in women and the prostate in men. Iodine is also vital for correct brain development and maintenance.

The other important aspect about iodine is that many substances have crept into our diets that prevent us from fully absorbing it. These include fluoride, chlorine, chloride, bromine, bromide, nitrates and nitrites. If fluoride is added to drinking water or toothpaste, then the iodine receptors, particularly within the thyroid, will have fluoride attached to them rather than iodine. A similar situation occurs with these other substances, all of which aggressively compete with iodine, displacing it from the cells. All of these substances have commonly been added to our food in one form or another to supposedly improve its quality or to make it safer to consume.

We also live with a much higher level of background radiation than in the past, especially since the advent of mobile phones and wi-fi. This causes a huge amount of electromagnetic interference, which disrupts the charge around our cell membranes and has profoundly negative effects upon the whole of our endocrine systems. Iodine is a natural antidote to radiation, but with a generally low intake of iodine and a high intake of iodine suppressors (fluoride, chlorine, etc.), we have little resistance to the many side effects of this man-made disruptive energy.

Iodine is also so important, particularly in the ovaries of women, in controlling the excessive synthetic oestrogens that have also crept into our food chain. These are found within the plastics in our environment, many of which are used in our food packaging. These substances leach into food and mimic our natural oestrogens, causing a huge hormonal imbalance that without sufficient iodine we can do little about.

Over the past hundred years many eminent doctors have become aware of this fact and have published their findings. These include Dr Max Gerson and Dr Derry, who both used iodine as an integral part of their successful treatment of cancer, and more recently Dr Abraham and Dr Brownstein.

We are currently living in a situation where the vibration of the Earth is consistently speeding up and, as we have seen throughout this book, we need to match our own vibration with that of the macrocosm. It is known that the speed of our metabolism is intrinsically linked to the thyroid and there are signs in our society that many people have an under-functioning thyroid. Lower-than-normal body temperature is a clear sign of this, but so too are the vast numbers of people taking synthetic thyroid hormones. The research by the above-mentioned doctors clearly points to iodine deficiency as the root cause of these problems.

Pharmaceutical companies have long been lobbying for a reduction in the recommended upper safety limits for all supplements and the proposed upper safety limit for iodine is 0.5 mg. This is 96 per cent below the minimum daily intake recommended by these physicians and clinicians who are have had so much success using iodine as an integral part of their treatment of a wide variety of health problems. If this becomes law I have no doubt that the spiralling levels of underactive thyroid, oestrogen-linked cancers and the many other health problems that have been shown to be linked to iodine deficiency will continue to rise. This of course is financially highly beneficial to the pharmaceutical companies which provide synthetic thyroid hormones, oestrogen-suppressing drugs and chemotherapy drugs, all of which have deeply worrying side effects.

It is my opinion that iodine is fundamental to human health and especially important in brain function. I see the suppression of iodine as an attempt to prevent us from fulfilling our potential and as a means of maintaining the status quo of the pharmaceutically driven medical profession. Every time I see a new piece of research that backs up the view that iodine is vital for health, I also see a piece of 'news' about how dangerous this natural substance is. Although I am not one for conspiracy theories, I clearly see that we are being given contradictory and confusing information and have to ask why. Once again the only answer is to take personal responsibility for discovering the truth for ourselves.

'The recommended daily amount of iodine for supplementation by clinicians of previous generations, that is 12.5–37.5 mg in the form of Lugol's solution, turns out to be the exact range of intake for sufficiency of the whole body, based on a recently developed loading test.'

Guy E. Abraham, MD, FACN

GLOSSARY

Acute illness: A short-lived illness requiring lots of energy.

Biochemical processes: Chemical and physio-chemical processes which occur within living organisms.

Bio-photon: A photon produced in the body by the collision of two free radicals.

Cell membrane: The outer boundary of a cell, which has major control over the cell's function. It is made of lipids and protein.

Chronic illness: A deep, stagnant illness which is more difficult to shift than an acute illness.

Electrolytes: The macro-minerals – sodium, potassium, calcium and magnesium.

Electron: A negatively charged subatomic particle, the primary carrier of electricity in solids.

Enzymes: Proteins produced by a living organism to act as a catalyst for a biochemical reaction.

Equinox: A time of equal day and night, when the sun is at right angles to the equator. Usually around 21 March and 21 September.

Ion: An atom or molecule with either a positive or negative charge.

Macrocosm: The bigger picture, the universe, the cosmos.

Metabolism: The chemical processes that occur within a living organism to maintain life.

Microbe: A micro-organism, especially a bacterium.

Microcosm: An encapsulation in miniature. The small encapsulation of the bigger picture (the macrocosm).

Micro-organism: A very small life form.

Microzymes: Living organisms contained in healthy cells which under certain circumstances could evolve into bacteria to instigate changes. They could then change back when balance had been created. Imperishable and in all forms of life (plant up to human). Béchamp considered them a basic constituent of life.

Nodal: A zero point. Current or voltage.

Permeable: Allowing liquids or gases to pass through.

pH: A measure of acidity or alkalinity.

Photon: Particle representing a quantum of light.

Polarity: The distinction between positive and negative.

Prostaglandins: A group of compounds with varying hormone-like effects working with the endocrine glands.

Suppressive treatment: Treatment preventing an expression by the person which would have led to an improvement in overall health and wellbeing.

RESOURCES

Chapter 1
Edward Bach, *Heal Thyself*, C.W. Daniel, 1996
Gregg Braden, *The Divine Matrix*, Hay House, 2006
Dr Henry Lindlahr, *The Philosophy of Natural Therapeutics*,
Lindlahr Publishing Co., 1936; reissued Vermilion, 2005

Chapter 2
Olof Alexandersson, *Living Water: Viktor Schauberger and
the Secrets of Natural Energy*, Turnstone Press, 1982
Dr F. Batmanghelidj, *Your Body's Many Cries for Water*,
Global Health Solutions, 1994
Herb Boynton, Mark F. McCarthy and Richard D. Moore,
The Salt Solution, Avery Publishing Group Inc., 2001
Martin L. Budd, *Low Blood Sugar*, Thorsons, 1981
Masaru Emoto, *The Hidden Messages in Water*, Beyond
Words Publishing, 2004
Sebastian Kneipp, *My Water Cure, 1891*; reissued Standard
Publications, Inc., 2007
Bruce Lipton, *The Biology of Belief*, Hay House, 2008
Yogi Ramacharaka, *The Hindu Yogi Practical Water Cure*,
Yogi Publication Society, 1937; reissued 2007

DVDs
The College of Natural Nutrition, *Human
Potential*, 2007

Chapter 3

Marco Bischof, *Biophotonen: Das Licht in unseren Zellen (Biophotons: The Light in our Cells, as yet untranslated into English)*, Zweitausendeins, 1996

Johanna Budwig, *Flax Oil as a True Aid Against Arthritis, Heart Infarction, Cancer and Other Diseases*, Apple Publishing Co. Ltd, 1994

Mary Enig, *Know Your Fats*, Bethesda Press, 2000

Mae-Wan Ho, *The Rainbow and the Worm*, World Scientific Publishing Co. Ltd, 1993

Annie Padden Jubb and David Jubb, *Secrets of an Alkaline Body*, North Atlantic Books, 2004

Bruce Lipton, *The Biology of Belief*, Hay House, 2008

Jeremy Narby, *The Cosmic Serpent*, Victor Gollancz, 1998

James L. Oschman, *Energy Medicine*, Churchill Livingstone, 2000

Roger Taylor, 'Free Radicals and the Wholeness of the Organism', *Nexus*, vol. 13, no. 3, April–May 2006

DVDs

The College of Natural Nutrition, *Light and Energy Centres* and *The Endocrine System: Utilisation of Oil and Light*, 2007

See also the work of Fritz-Albert Popp at the International Institute of Biophysics, Station Hombroich, Kapellener Strasse, D-41472 Neuss, Germany; www.lifescientists.de.

Chapter 4
Harriet Beinfield, *Between Heaven and Earth*,
Ballantine Books, Inc., 1992
Dianne M. Connelly, *Traditional Acupuncture*, The Centre
for Traditional Acupuncture, 1975
Russell Foster and Leon Kreitzman, *Rhythms of Life*,
Profile Books, 2005
Annie Padden Jubb and David Jubb, *Secrets of an Alkaline
Body*, North Atlantic Books, 2004
Johanna Paunegger and Thomas Poppe, *Moontime*, C.W.
Daniel Co. Ltd., 1995

DVDs
The College of Natural Nutrition, *Working with Natural
Rhythms: The Five Element Theory*, 2007

Chapter 5
Herman Aihara, *Acid and Alkaline*, George Ohsawa
Macrobiotic Foundation, 1980
Robin Bottomley, *You Don't Have to Feel Unwell*, Newleaf,
2000
Max Gerson, *A Cancer Therapy*, The Gerson Institute,
1958
Dr Henry Lindlahr, *The Philosophy of Natural Therapeutics*,
Lindlahr Publishing Co., 1936; reissued Vermilion, 2005

DVDs
The College of Natural Nutrition, *Hering's Law
of Cure: Acute and Chronic Disease*, 2007

Chapter 6

Nancy Appleton, *The Curse of Louis Pasteur,* Choice, 1999

Harriet Beinfield, *Between Heaven and Earth*, Ballantine Books, Inc., 1992

Robin Bottomley, *You Don't Have to Feel Unwell*, Newleaf, 2000

Dianne M. Connelly, *Traditional Acupuncture*, The Centre for Traditional Acupuncture, 1975

Christine Maggiore, *What If Everything You Thought You Knew About AIDS Was Wrong?,* Bridge of Love, 1996

Weston Price, *Nutrition and Physical Degeneration*, P. B. Hoeber, 1939; reissued Price Pottenger Nutrition, 2008

Janine Roberts, *Fear of the Invisible*, Impact Investigative Media Productions, 2008

DVDs

The College of Natural Nutrition, *Working with Natural Rhythms: The Five Element Theory*, 2007

The College of Natural Nutrition, *The Tubercular Taint: Bacterial and Viral Activity (Pasteur vs Béchamp)*, 2007

Chapter 7

Stage One

Dr F. Batmanghelidj, *Your Body's Many Cries for Water,* Global Health Solutions, 1994

James Braley and Ron Hoggan, *Dangerous Grains: Why Gluten Cereal Grains May Be Hazardous to your Health*, Avery Health Guides, 2003

Sally Fallon and Mary Enig, *Nourishing Traditions: The Cookbook that Challenges Politically Correct Nutrition and the Diet Dictocrats*, New Trends Publishing, Inc., 1999
Max Gerson, *A Cancer Therapy*, The Gerson Institute, 1958
Elaine Gottschall, *Breaking the Vicious Cycle: Intestinal Health Through Diet*, Kirkton Press Ltd, 1994
Doris Grant and Jean Joice, *Food Combining for Health*, Thorsons, 1984
Luke Jackson, *A User Guide to the GF/CF Diet for Autism, Asperger Syndrome and ADHD*, Jessica Kingsley Publishers, 2001

Stage Two
Dr Johanna Budwig, *Flax Oil as a True Aid Against Arthritis, Heart Infarction, Cancer and Other Diseases*, Apple Publishing Co. Ltd, 1994
Mary Enig, *Know Your Fats*, Bethesda Press, 2000
Valerie Gennari Cooksley, *Seaweed*, Steward, Tabori and Chang, Inc., 2007
Patrick Holford and Dr James Braly, *The H Factor*, Piatkus Books, 2003
Frank Orthoefer, *Lecithin and Health*, Vital Health Publishing, 2004

Stage Three
Herb Boynton, Mark F. McCarthy and Richard D. Moore, *The Salt Solution*, Avery Publishing Group Inc., 2001
David Brownstein, MD, *Iodine: Why You Need It*, Alternative Medical Press, 2008

Carolyn Dean, *The Miracle of Magnesium,* Random House, Inc., 2003

Carl Pfeiffer, *Zinc and Other Micronutrients*, Keats Publishing, Inc., 1978

DVDs

The College of Natural Nutrition, *The Three Stages of Treatment*, 2007

Chapter 8
DVDs

The College of Natural Nutrition, *How to Take a Case History*, 2007

Chapter 9

J. W. Armstong, *The Water of Life: A Treatise on Urine Therapy*, True Health Publishing Company, 1951; reissued Vermilion, 2005

Martha M. Christy, *Your Own Perfect Medicine*, Future Med, 1994

Max Gerson, *A Cancer Therapy*, The Gerson Institute, 1958

William A. McGarey, *The Oil That Heals,* ARE Press, 1994

—, *Edgar Cayce and the Palma Christi*, ARE Press, 1967; reissued 1992

M. T. Morter, *Correlative Urinalysis: The Body Knows Best,* Best Research, 1988

Coen Van Der Kroon, *The Golden Fountain: The Complete Guide to Urine Therapy*, Gateway Books, 1995

DVDs
The College of Natural Nutrition, *Natural Nutrition Techniques*, 2007

Appendix II
David Brownstein, MD, *Iodine: Why You Need It*, Alternative Medical Press, 2008
David M. Derry, MD, PhD, *Breast Cancer and Iodine*, Trafford Publishing, 2001
Max Gerson, *A Cancer Therapy*, The Gerson Institute, 1958

Hay House Titles of Related Interest

The 8th Chakra, by Jude Currivan PhD

Biology of Belief, by Bruce Lipton

Fractal Time, by Gregg Braden

How Your Mind Can Heal Your Body,
by David R. Hamilton PhD

Love Thyself, by Masaru Emoto

Your Secret Laws of Power, by Alla Svirinskaya

About the Author

Barbara Wren has been teaching and lecturing for the past 27 years, showing people a different approach to healing through nutrition and healing techniques. She has been practising for 35 years and has always believed that the empowerment of the individual through contacting their own inner wisdom is the only true way back to wholeness and happiness within the universal laws and rhythms.

The uniqueness of her College of Natural Nutrition approach is always at the leading edge of healing the body so that it can dance with the universal rhythms and respond positively to ongoing changes.

For further information about Barbara and her work, please go to www.natnut.co.uk.

Notes

Notes

Notes